Understanding and Managing Change in Healthcare

Understanding and Managing Change in Healthcare

A Step-by-Step Guide

Jaqui Hewitt-Taylor

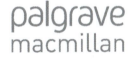

First published 2013 by
PALGRAVE MACMILLAN

Palgrave Macmillan in the UK is an imprint of Macmillan Publishers Limited, registered in England, company number 785998, of Houndmills, Basingstoke, Hampshire RG21 6XS.

Palgrave Macmillan in the US is a division of St Martin's Press LLC, 175 Fifth Avenue, New York, NY 10010.

Palgrave Macmillan is the global academic imprint of the above companies and has companies and representatives throughout the world.

Palgrave® and Macmillan® are registered trademarks in the United States, the United Kingdom, Europe and other countries.

ISBN 978–1–137–02276–9

This book is printed on paper suitable for recycling and made from fully managed and sustained forest sources. Logging, pulping and manufacturing processes are expected to conform to the environmental regulations of the country of origin.

A catalogue record for this book is available from the British Library.

A catalog record for this book is available from the Library of Congress.

To my eight-year-old son John, who finds the idea of change unnecessary

Contents

Figures

1

Introduction

What Is Change?

One of the few certainties we have is that we will all experience change during our lives. The changes that we encounter are sometimes so small or peripheral to us that we hardly notice them, whilst others are major events that affect almost every part of our lives. These changes may be planned, unplanned, our choice, or something that is imposed on us, and we may see them as working in our favour, or to our disadvantage. Some people enjoy change, and love the challenge of new circumstances or situations, whilst others find it disconcerting. However, the size, impact, and perceived benefit of any change, as well as the individual's natural response to change, will influence whether they see a particular situation as a positive opportunity, or a threat.

Change is also an almost guaranteed part of working life. The reasons for it, its extent, effect on individuals and organisations, people's attitudes to change in general, their perception of a particular change, and the way change is introduced, all influence whether it is welcomed or opposed. The complexity of the interactions between all these aspects of change and people's responses to it mean that the way change is managed merits considerable thought and planning. Sometimes the challenges that a change occasions seem out of proportion to its size: what appears to be a very small change can attract great antagonism, whilst other apparently more complex or major changes are achieved with relative ease. This is often because the way change is introduced and what the new way of working means to people are just as influential in their acceptance of it as the practicalities of what needs to be done differently (Parkin 2009: 160). A fairly common thing to hear about attempts to change practice is, 'It wasn't so much that we didn't think it was a good idea, we just didn't like the way it was done.' Managing the people aspects of change well greatly increases the chance of an innovation succeeding, rather than being a good idea that should have worked, but didn't (Schifalacqua et al. 2009, McLean 2011). However, in order to manage something effectively, it is useful to know what it is that is being managed. The term 'change' therefore merits definition.

> *How change is managed is as likely to influence its success as the value of the innovation itself.*

Change has been described as a process of moving from one identifiable state to another (Quattrone and Hopper 2001). A well-known illustration of the process of change draws an analogy with an ice cube melting, changing shape, and refreezing into a new shape (Lewin 1951). The initial frozen ice cube represents what was happening before anything changed; the process of the ice cube melting symbolises the stage at which change was suggested, people considered it, and began to accept the idea; the newly shaped ice denotes things beginning to change, and the old way gradually ceasing to exist. Finally, refreezing corresponds to the new way becoming accepted as the established way of doing things. Other descriptions of change tend to follow the same principle, of a process of movement from one state of being to another. Guy and Gibbons (2003), for example, describe how change involves people moving from accepting their current situation to becoming motivated to want things to be different, adjusting the way things are, and the new situation becoming the norm. Change is, therefore, generally seen to involve an alteration of some aspect of a state of being, in order to create a new state. Planning change is essentially about planning what the new state of being will be, how to get there, how you will know that you have arrived, and how you will make sure that you stay there (if you should) or move on, rather than going back to where you were before.

> *Planning change is like planning a journey: it should include not just where people will go, and how they will get there, but what might make them want to make the journey, and stay there once they have arrived.*

Change and Practice Development

Managing change effectively is thought to be a key part of developing practice, as the latter generally involves changing some aspect of the way things are done, perceived, or both (International Council of Nurses 2009, Reid and Weller 2010, World Health Organization 2010). However, change per se does not improve or develop practice: that depends on whether what changes results in improvements for anyone. In terms of developing practice, the question is not 'Has anything changed?' but 'Has anything changed which has contributed to improving practice?'

There are different approaches to developing practice, but the most commonly cited distinctions involve whether practice development is seen as a technical process, or as a way of enabling people, as well as discrete elements of practice, to change. The former approach is often described as technical practice development, whilst the latter has been described as emancipatory (Wilson and McCormack 2006), or transformational, practice development (Walsh et al. 2011). In what is termed technical practice development, changing or developing practice primarily concerns technical or procedural change. Here, a new way of doing something is identified, and people are taken through a process of learning about it, and gaining the skills needed to alter the way they work. The focus is on the particular task, and the new way of carrying it out: any other development of the individuals involved, or the service in question, is an additional bonus (Manley and McCormack 2003). For example, if an intensive care unit is experiencing problems with the number of arterial lines that are becoming dislodged, a new way of securing arterial lines may be found; everyone will be taught how to secure arterial lines this way and, if it is a better method, there will be less problems with arterial lines and care will be improved. However, apart from accepting that this way of securing arterial lines is better, and learning how to secure the lines, those involved will not have developed their way of thinking particularly, and the change in practice ends with the new way of securing arterial lines becoming established as a good thing that everyone should do. The benefit of technical practice development is that a very specific aspect of practice is improved.

An alternative approach to practice development is to view it as an emancipatory or transformational process (hence the terms 'emancipatory practice development' and 'transformational practice development'). In these approaches, the central focus is on enabling practitioners to reflect on their practice, challenge this, and develop the skills and confidence to design and trial new ways of working, with the aim of improving care (Wilson and McCormack 2006). An emancipatory or transformational approach to practice development often still requires technical inputs because new ways of working frequently require specific skills and knowledge to be developed. However, the process involved in changing practice enables and empowers individuals to question and alter the way things are done, and to change the way they see themselves and their practice. They have as their conclusion not just specific changes or improvements in how particular aspects of care are carried out, but a workforce that seeks to constantly question, refine, and develop practice (Wilson and McCormack 2006). An emancipatory approach to practice development might be seen when someone notices that there is a problem with the way arterial lines are secured, wonders whether there is a better way to secure them, raises the issue with colleagues, looks into alternatives, and discusses these with the team; and the team reaches a decision and tries a new method. If this new way of securing arterial lines is shown to work better, it becomes an accepted practice on the unit. On the surface, this process has exactly the same outcome as technical practice development: a better way of securing arterial lines is identified, lines are secured more effectively, and patient care is improved. The difference is not so much in where things end in relation to a specific procedure, but in the journey to getting there, and what is learned and developed en route. In emancipatory practice development, skills are developed and a particular aspect of care is improved, and so are individuals. Those who are directly involved in delivering care instigate and facilitate the process of changing the way things are done, and, by their involvement in the process, develop the habits of mind to question what is happening, think about what could be improved, and acquire the skills and confidence to try new approaches. By developing the way people think, as well as refining specific aspects of practice, emancipatory practice development creates a culture in which innovation is nurtured (Manley and McCormack 2003). This ultimately means that developing practice becomes a natural and continuous process; for example, having successfully developed a better way of securing arterial lines, people may begin to think about how central lines are kept in place, and if this could be improved.

Transformational practice development has commonalities with emancipatory practice development, in that the people involved in changing the way things are done also develop personally (Walsh et al. 2011). However, in this approach those involved learn to be critically reflective about themselves, their workplace, and their practice, including the assumptions, values, and priorities, which underpin these. From this critical reflection, as well as individuals' development of their ability to change practice, a transformation of their thinking about themselves and their work can develop, which alters not only discrete aspects of practice, but how practice as a whole and the values on which it is based are viewed (Dewing 2010, Walsh et al. 2011).

Approaches to Practice Development

Technical: focuses on changing technical or procedural aspects of practice;

Emancipatory: focuses on enabling practitioners to reflect on their practice, challenge this, and develop the skills and confidence to change practice;

> **Approaches to Practice Development**   *continued*
>
> *Transformational*: focuses on individuals and teams becoming critically reflective about the assumptions, values, and priorities that underpin their work and their workplace, and from this developing innovations in practice.

Whilst no one approach to developing practice will fit every instance where change is needed, the ideal approach to change is to see it as a part of, or a step towards, emancipatory or transformational practice development, where individuals and services are engaged in a culture of constant learning and evolution. However, not every situation is immediately amenable to this way of working. Sometimes change is required of an organisation, and those within in, rather than being something that evolves from practitioners' reflective activities. In addition, not every individual or team is accustomed to, or has embraced, a way of thinking that is compatible with this approach (Cameron and Green 2009: 83). Emancipatory or transformational practice development, however desirable, may, therefore, not always be possible in their pure or most highly developed form. Nevertheless, working within the ethos or principles of emancipatory practice development, or towards developing a transformational approach to developing practice, is generally desirable. The focus throughout this book is on working with the people involved in and affected by change, so as to maximise their participation in, ownership of, and development through new ways of working. The emphasis throughout is predominantly on the people aspects of change management.

There is no one 'right' way to approach developing practice. Noting where your team is now, and planning what you hope to achieve in the short and long term can help you to decide which approach is the most appropriate.

People and Product in Change

Paton and McCalman (2008: 138–142) suggest that change may be concerned with issues that exist on a continuum from mechanistic processes to people-centred matters. In purely mechanistic change, as the name suggests, the only thing that needs to be considered is changing a mechanism or procedure. People-centred change, in contrast, is concerned with human factors such as interactions, values, and priorities. Although change can be described as existing on this continuum, few changes in healthcare can really be placed at its mechanistic extreme, as almost every change requires people to be considered. Even if a proposed change in practice is something as apparently procedural as moving the intravenous fluids from one side of the store cupboard to the other, its successful execution may be heavily influenced by the people side. Moving bags of fluids to a new location is fairly easy, but convincing people that this is a good thing to do can be surprisingly hard or contentious. There may be a very good reason why the fluids are stored where they are, the person who put them there may feel offended about them being moved, and their friends may feel this on their behalf. If the person making the suggestion is relatively new in post, their action may be perceived to imply that they feel they can, without any good reason, change things that have worked well for years. A great deal of attention usually needs to be given to managing the people side of attempting to introduce any innovation in practice, because that is the part that is hardest to predict or get right, and which is most likely to scupper the best laid practical arrangements for change (McLean 2011). It is also the aspect of change that is likely to influence whether or not an innovation becomes a part of a route to emancipation or transformation. If the way change is handled disempowers or offends people, it is unlikely to become a part of a process that facilitates the development of a culture of emancipatory or transformational practice development.

Similarly, there are often seen as being two important and sometimes discrete aspects of change. One is the new way of working itself, and another is how people feel about this and how it affects them personally. Austin and Currie (2003) and McLean (2011) describe these two aspects as 'change' and 'transition'. They describe change as the external aspect of an alteration in the status quo: the observable things that happen or are done differently. This might be the more technical part of change, the part that concerns, for example, exactly where the bags of intravenous fluids will now be stored. Transition, on the other hand, is about the emotional or psychological element of change: what people feel, experience, and see as important. How people feel about changing the place the intravenous fluids are stored, what happened the last time someone changed the location of the fluids, whether they see this as a necessary change or change for change's sake, whether it is viewed as a challenge to someone or something that they value, and how the individuals concerned manage these feelings. Even if a new way of doing something does not seem to be a major change from current practice, if the transition for the individuals involved is significant, there needs to be considerable input into the process of managing the people side of change for it to be a success. This may explain why some changes that seem minor are very difficult to achieve: the change is easy, but the transition is complex or difficult.

For change to succeed, the practicalities and people elements need to be given equal attention.

Roles in Change Management

People can adopt a number of different roles in the process of change management, and various terms are used to denote these roles, including change leader, change agent, and change champion. The term 'change leader' usually refers to the person who will take overall control, charge of, and responsibility for the change process. They are often the person with the initial idea for change, but this may not always be the case. An 'ideas person' is not always a good or willing leader, or a person who is well suited to carrying a plan through. In addition, the person who takes on the overall leadership of a project may not be responsible for the day-to-day management of the minutiae of the activities that are necessary for change to take place.

Along with the term 'change leader', the term 'change agent' is often used to identify the person or people who will take a lead role in the day-to-day process of facilitating change (Cameron and Green 2009: 158, Schulenkorf 2010). Although they are responsible for the day-to-day implementation of the process of change, change agents may have no direct line of authority over those who are required to alter the way they work (Cameron and Green 2009: 158). Key qualities for successful change agents are described as including commitment to the new way of working, understanding of why it is happening, and the ability to enthuse others about it (Bennett 2003, Schulenkorf 2010). They usually need to be able to solve problems and make appropriate decisions, because they are the key people in the practical instigation of the new way of working (Bennett 2003). Perhaps, most importantly, they need 'people skills': the ability to build trust amongst those who need to change the way they work; communicate effectively with those involved in and affected by the change; and network advantageously with those who may not be directly involved in, but who have an influence over, the change happening (Schulenkorf 2010).

It is fairly unrealistic to expect one person to have all of these qualities and the time to achieve all these tasks. Not everyone who is good at enthusing people is a good decision-maker, not everyone who is good at inspiring trust in their immediate colleagues is good at enthusing people, and not everyone is in a position to spend all their time on a particular project; so more than one person often needs to be involved in leading or facilitating change. For change to be successful, the right people also need to be doing the right things. A key part of managing successful change is involving people to the greatest overall advantage, so that all the requisite roles and activities are covered, people are doing what they are good at and enjoy doing, and the workload is made realistic by it being spread across a group.

Roles Needed for Successful Change

Ideas people
Leader or leaders
Day-to-day facilitators
People who will support and champion change

The term 'change champion' has some overlaps with the term 'change agent', and the terms are sometimes used synonymously, although change champions do not usually fulfil all the roles required of a change agent. They are generally seen as being more closely involved in literally championing, or supporting and promoting, change and encouraging others to work in the new way on a day-to-day basis (Hendy and Barlow 2011). Roles that have been linked with change champions include educating, advocating, working with people to help them to accept innovation, and building relationships (Soo et al. 2009). If a change is being implemented across a whole organisation, change champions who will be pro-change representatives may be sought in each unit, ward, department, or team.

The important point in managing change is perhaps not so much what you call those who take on key roles, as knowing what aspects of the planning and implementation of change need to be covered, who should be involved, what their skills are, how these match the required roles, and how you can best involve and work with them to bring about change that will last.

Change requires people to take on various roles and responsibilities. A key skill in planning change is determining the best person for each role.

Overview of the Rest of the Book

The intention of this book is to describe the journey through the process of changing practice, from identifying a need for change to publicising its outcomes. Each chapter is based on a scenario or scenarios, which are used to illustrate the main issues covered in that chapter, and is followed by a case study that illustrates the key issues that have been discussed. At the end of each chapter, there is a section of guided work, which can be completed alone, or with colleagues.

Chapter 2 discusses why a change in practice might be proposed, and possible ways of approaching change in three different situations: one where a problem has arisen in practice, one where a new policy is being imposed on a service, and one where a piece of research has made someone consider changing the way things are done. Chapter 3 explores creating and maintaining motivation for adopting new practice, including approaches to encouraging others to change their practice, identifying the aims and objectives of change, involving the right people, and taking into account personal and organisational priorities in change. Chapter 4 looks at planning change, starting with assessing the factors that are likely to drive and restrain change, and individual and corporate readiness for change. It then progresses through the steps required to create an achievable plan for change. Chapter 5 discusses resistance and barriers to change and highlights their benefits as well as challenges, before considering specific aspects of resistance, and ways in which these may be managed. Chapter 6 focuses on the point at which planning is complete and new practice is rolled out. With regard to the immediate practicalities and necessities of this stage, it discusses how motivation can be maintained, different levels of support managed, and setbacks or alterations to the original plan accommodated. Chapter 7 discusses multidisciplinary aspects of change. It outlines the different ways in which disciplines may work together, why multidisciplinary involvement in change is often necessary in healthcare, and how to decide which disciplines and individuals from these need to be involved in a particular innovation.

Having reached the point at which change is rolled out in the first half of the book, the latter chapters discuss what happens after that point. Chapter 8 outlines the process of designing and conducting evaluation of change and locates evaluation at the beginning of the next stage of practice development rather than as the end point of a stand-alone activity. Chapter 9 discusses the importance of learning from change, which has not gone to plan, or not achieved its expected outcomes, and the potential benefits that may still be derived from such situations. Chapter 10 discusses the challenge of maintaining new practice after the initial implementation phase. It highlights the risk of slipping back into old ways after change appears to have taken place and suggests some ways of avoiding this and maintaining enthusiasm for, and commitment to, the new way of working. Chapter 11 discusses the importance of, and possible approaches to, disseminating new evidence derived from changed practice, including ideas on how to share new knowledge locally, nationally and internationally.

The book aims to provide a practice-focused, step-by-step guide to planning and managing the process of change. However, there is no one right way to manage change: it depends on the situation, people, and nature of the change involved (Cameron and Green 2009: 135). The best way to manage change depends on what you are changing, why you are changing it, and who is involved. Because the people aspects of change are usually the most important, there is no one fail-safe protocol or process that can be followed, in all situations, with an absolute guarantee of success. This book outlines some of the principles that increase the chances of change being effective. However, none will always work in every situation. Life and the people in it aren't like that.

2

Identifying a Need for Change

Chapter Learning Outcomes

After studying this chapter, the reader will be able to:

- Use appropriate approaches to identify and analyse problems in practice
- Consider how control and choice for those affected by change can be maximised even in imposed change
- Identify various types of evidence that might inform change and their relative value
- Understand the principles of evaluating evidence for use in practice.

Summary

This chapter explores three situations where a change in practice might be proposed: because of a problem that creates a risk to patient safety, because of a new policy, or because there is evidence that a better approach to care provision may exist.

The section on changing practice in response to a problem includes a discussion of problem identification and analysis strategies and how these processes can assist in identifying achievable and relevant solutions.

The section concerning change that is required because of a new protocol explores how the reason for the change, the degree of choice available in its implementation, and the manner in which this is negotiated with and communicated to staff can affect its likely success.

The section about change that is proposed because of evidence that something could be done better includes discussion of types of evidence, evaluation of evidence, and deciding on how applicable to a particular practice situation the available evidence is.

The first stage of bringing about any change in practice is to decide what needs to change, and why (Hall and Hord 2011: 43). Chapter 1 suggested that the ideal way for change to be initiated is for practitioners to look at and reflect on the way things are done and decide what could be improved (Wilson and McCormack 2006). However, this is not always how things happen: there are times when change is imposed on a workplace to fit with national or local organisational strategy, structure, or policy. On other occasions, change is required because an incident or adverse event means that something has to be done to avoid the problem recurring.

Identifying how and why a need for change has arisen, and how this may affect acceptance of it, is an important first step in planning the best way to manage the process of changing practice. This chapter explores three scenarios where implementing change is being planned: one in which change is needed because of a problem in practice, one where change is required because of a new protocol, and one in which change is being advocated because of an idea that someone has had for developing service provision.

A Problem in Practice

Jane is a deputy ward manager on a medical ward that specialises in rheumatology. It was recently brought to the ward manager's attention that the number of falls amongst patients on the ward had increased. He was required to look into how falls would be reduced and to produce a plan of action to improve the situation. Jane was asked to take a lead role in this, and the ward manager suggested that she should revisit the form used to assess the risk of patients falling. Other staff also told Jane their views on the causes of the problem: poor staffing levels and increasing numbers of seriously ill patients, often medical outliers, whose care needs left the nurses unable to supervise the less acutely ill patients (who tended to be those who had falls) adequately. The general feeling was that unless the ward had 'decent staffing levels' nothing could be done to improve matters. However, there was a requirement to show that changes would be made to address this issue, and additional staffing did not appear to be an option.

When a solution to a problem is being sought, finding the cause of the apparent problem is the cornerstone of designing an effective solution. Otherwise, a change that addresses the problem's effect, but not its cause, may be instigated (van Meijel et al. 2004, Parkin 2009: 147–149). On Jane's ward, the apparent problem was an increased number of falls. However, to find an effective solution to this, she needed to know what was causing the rising number of falls, and to design an intervention that would address this.

Problem Identification

Before starting to explore the cause of a problem, it is useful to identify whether the presenting issue is really problematic (Garavaglia 2008, Okes 2008). Jane began her investigation into the increasing incidence of falls by trying to identify whether there really was a rise in the number of falls on her ward. She felt that this probably was the case, but there had been three complaints from relatives of patients who had fallen in the past two weeks, and she wanted to be sure that an isolated cluster of incidents was not clouding the real picture of trends in falls. To get a more accurate impression of what was happening, she checked the incident reports over the past six months, and compared these to the same six-month period from the previous year, to see if the number of falls-related reports had risen. This comparison showed a marked increase in falls-related reports. She also checked the statistics on bed usage at the times in question to determine whether the increase in falls was related to increased patient numbers, which might naturally increase the number of falls. Bed occupancy per se had not increased, but patient turnover was more rapid than it had been the previous year, and there were more seriously ill and outlying patients housed on the ward. This seemed to corroborate the suggestion that staff had made about their workload having changed. Jane checked the rotas and found that the number of nurses on each shift was approximately the same as it had been the previous year, but the proportion of bank and agency staff being used to maintain this level had risen. Her investigation showed that falls were an increasing problem, and that this might be associated with changes in staffing, the type of patients, and dependency levels on the ward.

Problems in Practice: Things to Consider

What do people say the problem is?
Does everyone see this as the problem?
What evidence is there to show that there is a problem?
When and where does the problem occur most often?
How significant is the problem?

It is also useful to look at when and where a problem occurs, to see if this provides any information about its cause (Okes 2008). Jane looked at the timings of falls: the highest number happened during handover times, and very few occurred during visiting hours. The majority of falls also involved patients who were housed in the lower dependency and less easily observed areas of the ward. Those whose falls had been recorded on incident forms were almost always noted to have been assessed as being at risk of falling. This led Jane to think that the problem was not about the assessment of the risk of falls happening, but what was done with that information. It also made her think about the group of patients who were most affected, and the timing of falls, which was useful in her later problem analysis and consideration of solutions (see Figure 2.1).

Although any problem in practice matters, most workplaces have a number of competing demands on their time and resources, and, even if a problem does exist, a decision has to be made about the priority that it should be afforded. Noting how often a problem occurs, as well as where and when it happens, helps to gauge how serious, or urgent, addressing it is (Okes 2008). Although Jane had found that there were more falls on the ward than there had been during the previous year, she also noted their frequency, to see if this was within what might be considered an acceptable limit, or whether the problem merited urgent intervention.

Jane's investigation clarified that a problem did exist, and merited priority attention. It also highlighted factors that might contribute to the problem. However, to be able to decide how to change practice in a way that would address the causes of the problem, the situation needed to be analysed further (Okes 2008).

The first stage of changing practice in response to a problem is to check whether there really is a problem, exactly what the problem is, and how significant it is.

Problem Analysis

In order to develop her ideas about a solution, or solutions, to the problem of the increased number of falls on her ward, Jane now needed to establish exactly how or why each circumstance that her initial investigation had linked to falls contributed to them, and whether there were any other contributory factors that her initial investigation had missed. When you are looking at problems in your own workplace, it can be hard to completely put aside your assumptions, and personal opinions, about the situation (Paton and McCalman 2008: 240). Jane aimed to gain as objective and thorough a view of the situation as she could by using a process or tool, which made her think about all the possible causes of the problem she was unpicking, and why they resulted in falls. The process of problem analysis, which is aimed at identifying the cause, or causes, of a problem can be useful in this respect (van Bokhoven et al. 2003, European Commission 2004).

There are a variety of problem analysis tools that Jane could have used, but she chose one known as the Five Whys approach. This approach explores the cause or causes of a problem by repeatedly asking why something happens or exists. It begins with a statement of what the problem is, and the first why that is asked is: 'Why does this happen?' or 'Why has this happened?' This is followed by repeatedly asking 'why' until the root cause or causes of the problem become clear. These causes can then be used as a basis for considering solutions. The number five is an approximate value: the principle is that it is necessary to ask why until no further why questions would be helpful (Latino 2004). How the whys are recorded depends on individual preference, but they are often presented as a table or a fishbone diagram.

The problem that Jane identified was an increase in falls. She began her Five Whys analysis with the statement: 'There are an increased number of falls amongst patients who have been assessed as being at risk of falling.' This led to her first why: 'Why has this happened?' From this, she documented her subsequent 'whys' in tabular format, as shown in Figure 2.1. Alongside the answer to each 'why', it is useful to note the source of evidence that informs the response, so that the certainty with which this is known can be gauged (Latino 2004). Jane noted her sources of evidence on the Five Whys table; for example, 'staff rota' against how she knew about staffing levels and skill mix.

Other tools or methods that Jane could have used include a fishbone diagram (Ishikawa), Problem Tree analysis, or the Seven S model. A fishbone diagram may be used in its own right, or as a way of representing the Five Whys analysis. In this approach, problems and their possible causes are depicted as a fish skeleton: the head of the fish represents the problem, and contributory factors are shown as the spines (Iles and Cranfield 2004). When a fishbone is used as a way of documenting the Five Whys analysis, the spines are identified by asking the initial 'why' with smaller bones added to the spines as each original 'why' is explored in more detail. If Jane had used a fishbone Diagram to document her Five Whys analysis, it might have looked something like Figure 2.2.

Problem Tree analysis (also referred to as situational analysis) uses the image of a tree to structure and illustrate the exploration of a problem. Like the Five Whys analysis and fishbone diagram, Problem Tree analysis aims to distinguish a problem, its causes and effects, and thus to enable solutions that address the cause or causes of a problem to be devised (Hovland 2005). The process begins with a starter problem being documented (for example, an increased number of falls) and from this related problems or issues are identified. The issues causing the starter problem are placed below it, and become the tree's roots, and those that are the effects or consequences of it are put above it, and become the branches (European Commission 2004). Each time an issue is identified, the question: 'What causes that?' is posed, so that cause and effect are distinguished and each statement can be placed

Why has this happened?				
Current staffing levels and skill mix are not adequate to enable staff to supervise all the patients	The current staffing level is not adequate to enable staff to meet all the patients' needs	The mix of patients on the ward makes it difficult to provide for all their care needs	Patients who fall are often in bays which are less well supervised than others	Falls often happen during staff handover times (evidence: incident reports state time of incident)
Why?	Why?	Why?	Why?	Why?
Many staff are not familiar with the ward, and therefore cannot take on as heavy a workload as permanent staff can (evidence: discussion with staff)	The overall dependency level of patients on the ward is higher than that in previous years, but staffing levels are the same (evidence: ward dependency score data and rotas)	The ward has patients from an increasing range of different medical specialities, which increases staff workloads (evidence: admissions book and discussion with staff)	They tend to be the less acutely ill patients and are housed in lower dependency areas (evidence: incident forms state patient location)	During handover one nurse is always away from the ward area
Why?	Why?	Why?	Why?	Why?
A lot of bank and agency staff are being used, who are often unfamiliar with the ward (evidence: staff rotas)	The trend for more care to be provided at home means that those who are in hospital are more acutely ill, but bed numbers, occupancy, and staffing levels on the ward are still the same (evidence: staff roats and ward dependency scores)	Pressure on beds means that there are a significant number of medical outliers on the ward, and this makes care provision more difficult and time consuming for staff (evidence: ward admission book and discussions with staff)	High observation areas are allocated to patients at risk of acute deterioration (evidence: observation of ward processes)	Handover happens in the office
Why?	Why?	Why?	Why?	Why?

Figure 2.1 Five Whys analysis

There are a lot of shifts that cannot be covered by permanent staff (evidence: staff rotas)	The pressure on beds throughtout the Trust remains high because two wards have closed	Staff are less familiar with the care needs and treatments required by outliers (evidence: discussion with staff)	Acutely ill patients are usually deemed to need the greatest supervision	Walk round handovers and handovers at the nurses' station were found to be constantly interrupted (evidence: ward meeting notes)
Why?	Why?	Why?	Why?	Why?
Two staff are on long-terms sick leave and one is on maternity leave. They cannot be replaced (evidence: staff rotas)	Although beds have closed, those which remains are constantly in demand	Many staff have worked on this ward for a long time and have a specialist interest in rheumatology, not other areas of medical nursing (evidence: staff profiles)	Potentially life-threatening issues take priority	Staff were perceived to be available and often interrupted or called away during alternative approaches to handover (evidence: ward meeting notes)
Possible solutions: employ a higher ratio of temporary staff or close beds	Possible solution: increase staffing levels or alter bed allocation	Possible solutions: in service training on the conditions most commonly encountered in outliers/rotation of staff to other wards to learn about other specialities	Possible solution: more supervision available in low dependency areas by increased staffing levels/move patients at risk of falling to high dependency areas	Possible solution: retry alternative approaches to handovers/ increase staffing levels at handover times

Figure 2.1 (Continued)

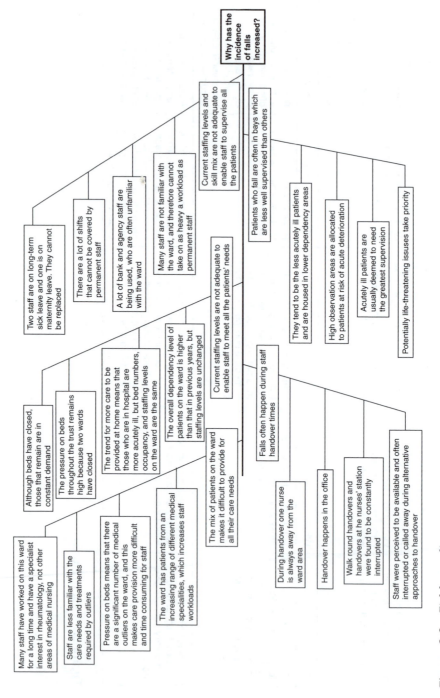

Figure 2.2 Fishbone diagram

appropriately in the overall picture of the problem situation. If Jane had used this approach, her diagram might have looked something like that shown in Figure 2.3.

The Seven S model (Iles and Cranfield 2004, Cameron and Green 2009: 122) is a way of mapping out the key elements of a team or organisation, what roles they might play in a problem that has been identified, and how they interact with each other. The elements represented by the Seven Ss are Strategy, Structure, Systems, Staff, Style of management, Shared beliefs/values, and Skills. If Jane had used this approach, she might have thought about what staff were needed to prevent patients from falling, what skills these staff needed to have, and whether these were currently available. Any one of the 'Ss' may fall into more than one category: staff experience or expertise, for instance, might fall within 'skills' and 'staffing'. It is also useful to map the Ss against each other to see how one may influence the rest. For instance, Jane might have asked, 'Does the structure of the ward make best use of the existing staff?' This approach can be used as an aid to thinking about all the aspects of a problem, and how they may affect, and be affected by, each other.

Although the process of problem analysis can be very useful to give an overview of and indications about the causes and effects of a situation, no one approach can, of itself, include or explain all the complexities of every aspect of a problem (European Commission 2004). Each approach to problem analysis has strengths and limitations, and it may be useful to carry out more than one analysis of a problem, using different tools, to gain more perspectives. For example, the Five Whys analysis and fishbone diagram do not easily allow the links between causes to be shown, and rely on the cause, or causes, of a problem being able to be fairly neatly articulated. They also tend to suggest that a clear root cause or causes that can be directly linked to a solution exist, which is not always the case (Latino 2004). The Problem Tree analysis can show more links between the potentially complex and interrelated causes of a problem situation, although illustrating their real complexity will always be difficult to achieve. A limitation of many problem analysis tools, including the Five Whys, Fishbone, and Problem Tree approaches, is that they do not give prompts about what it might be useful to consider in analysing the problem: one aspect of the increasing incidence of falls that Jane's problem analysis did not include was staff attitudes and values, and whether they saw preventing falls as an important issue. This was alluded to in terms of the statement that: 'Potentially life threatening situations take priority,' but did not explore staff or organisational beliefs about the importance of preventing falls, or the priority given to supervising lower dependency areas of the ward. This might have been more comprehensively identified by using a tool that provided specific prompts, such as

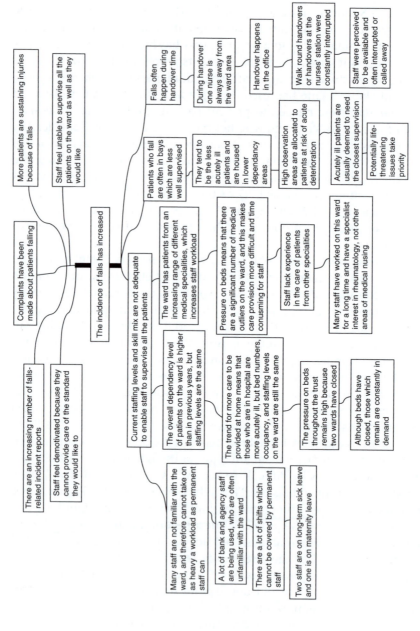

Figure 2.3 Problem Tree analysis

the Seven S model, where shared beliefs is highlighted as an element to consider. However, a downside of the Seven S model is that it may not guide the questioner to look in as much depth at the root causes of a problem as some other approaches, and may not create such a clear pathway to considering solutions. The problem analysis tools available are intended to guide and enable those confronted with problem situations to unpick and consider the causes and effects involved, but they cannot, of themselves, fully identify the complexities of, or solutions to, any particular practice problem.

Analysing a problem should enable its causes, rather than its effects, to be identified.

Finding Solutions

The findings from Jane's analysis suggested that there were several issues, which contributed to falls, and more than one possible solution. However, any solution had to be achievable. The obvious solutions of improving staffing levels, reducing the number of outlying patients, or relocating beds were unlikely to be achievable. Providing more training and experience in other areas of practice to increase staff confidence would take time to achieve, and staff would have to be free to attend training or rotations. Given the current staffing difficulties, this was also unlikely to be achievable in the immediate future.

Handover times seemed to present the highest risk of falls. Different approaches to handover, which made more staff available on the ward, had been trialled, and although they could be revisited, the opposition to them after the trial had been recent and strenuous. So this option, whilst potentially valuable in the longer term, did not seem achievable at present. Ideally, perhaps, more staff could be made available at handover times, but this was a busy time hospital-wide, and additional staffing cover was therefore unlikely. Falls were most common in patients not only who had been identified as being at risk of falling, but who were housed in the low observation area of the ward. Moving patients who were identified as being at risk of falls to high observation areas was unlikely to be possible, as the pressure on the high observation beds would remain.

The Five Why analysis had not really offered any solutions to the problem, but it had enabled Jane to see that staff being unable to supervise the lower dependency areas of the ward, particularly at key times, seemed to be the major issue. She noted that few falls happened during visiting times, and thought that this might be because someone was available to notice when a patient wanted something, and to call a nurse, which was not otherwise always possible, especially if the patient concerned had difficulty in using the call system, or communicating. She wondered whether using hospital volunteers to provide general supervision of the low dependency areas, especially during 'high risk' times such as the handover period, or introducing open visiting would be options worth exploring, so as to have more people around, especially at key times.

Jane realised that, for any new way of working to succeed, she would need the rest of the ward staff to see changing the way things were done as important, and to be prepared to work with whatever solution was decided upon. To achieve this, she wanted staff to engage in exploring the problem, suggesting and owning solutions to it, rather than these being dictated (Paton and McCalman 2008: 29, Hall and Hord 2011: 148). She had felt it necessary to gather facts about what was happening, carry out her own analysis of the problem, and have some information and ideas to offer. However, having done this, she now planned to have a discussion with the rest of the ward staff, using the Five Whys approach to analysing the problem, to gain their perceptions. This would give them the chance to engage in the process, offer their perspectives, and suggest alternative solutions.

Analysing problems will not immediately provide a solution, but should mean that solutions that address the cause, not the effect, can be designed.

In this case, thinking about changing how things were done was necessary because of an identified problem in practice. In other cases, change may be required because new policies, protocols, or systems are being introduced.

Change in Response to a New Policy or Protocol

Andrew is a team leader of a community nursing team. He recently received details of a new protocol that was being introduced for the management and administration of drugs via long-term intravenous catheters. When Andrew read this, he realised that his staff were unlikely to welcome it. The team had three patients who used these devices, and, as far as Andrew was aware, no problems had ever been reported with the lines, how they were cared for, or accessed. The new protocol seemed more complex than current practice, and required a procedure that his team was not familiar with to be followed. Although Andrew guessed that this innovation would not be popular, the information sent with the protocol indicated that it was to be implemented immediately.

Unless people are convinced that a new way of working is needed, and of how it might improve things, they are unlikely to be keen to change their working practice (Hodges 2008, Weiner 2009). Andrew felt that this was the major issue that would present when he asked his team to adopt the new protocol: why the request was being made, and its possible benefits, were not clear to him. As a result, he would find it difficult to convince anyone else of the importance of changing the way they worked. He therefore sought more information, so that he could decide how to manage the situation.

The Basis of the Policy or Protocol

Whilst people usually require a good reason to change the way they work, if they understand why a new way of working is being proposed, they are seldom as intrinsically opposed to change as is often supposed (Paton and McCalman 2008: 12). Before meeting with his staff to advise them of the new protocol, Andrew therefore wanted to find out why it had been introduced.

It transpired that other teams had experienced some adverse incidents with long-term intravenous catheters, including frequent blocking and line infections. Because of this, a new protocol had been devised, and then trailed by the team who had the largest number of patients with this type of line. They had given positive feedback on the changes, and their rates of infection and lines blockage had reduced. The Primary Care Trust (PCT) as a whole was therefore now going to adopt this approach. It became apparent that the other teams in the PCT had already had input about the new protocol, but that, for some reason, Andrew's team had not received the interim information about it.

This information helped Andrew to understand why the protocol had been devised. It also clarified why it had arrived, apparently without discussion, with a demand for immediate implementation. His enquiry enabled Andrew to begin to think about what would need to be put in place for his team to accept the new way of working, including the resources and training that would be necessary (Golden 2006, MacPhee and Suryaparkash 2012). The conversation also meant that those requiring the change in practice were made aware that his team had not been prepared for the new way of working, would probably not see it as necessary, and that this was likely to create problems with its implementation (Weiner 2009). This gave Andrew an opportunity to initiate discussions about how the new protocol could be rolled out with his team, so as to overcome some of the likely barriers to it being accepted.

If people understand the reason for a change in practice being requested, they are more likely to accept it.

The Nature of Change

When any change is proposed, it is useful to think about the effect it will have on those required to do it (Scott et al. 2003, Golden 2006). As Chapter 1 identified, change may exist anywhere on a continuum between being purely mechanistic or people centred (Paton ad McCalman 2008: 21–25). In this case, whilst the practicalities of the protocol for managing long-term intravenous catheters appeared to be what was to change, the people aspect was, as is often the case, equally, and probably more, significant than the technical aspects (McLean 2011). Staff would move from doing something that they were familiar with, where the process and expectations were known, to territory that was unfamiliar to them, and those whom they worked with. This was likely to create feelings of uncertainty, or anxiety, for staff and patients. They might also feel angry or resentful that they were placed in this position, and appeared not to have been valued enough to be consulted about the change in how lines were managed. As Chapter 1 identified, change will almost always involve what Austin and Currie (2003) and McLean (2011) term transition: people's feelings about and responses to it, and how it is introduced, as well as the process or procedure that alters. Andrew felt it likely that the people centred, or transitional, elements of the new way of working, rather than the new way of managing the lines itself, would make his team disinclined to adopt it.

Having considered these points, Andrew discussed with those who had instigated the protocol how he could adapt the plans for implementing it, in order to gain his team's co-operation.

If you are asked to implement a change in practice that you feel your colleagues are likely to oppose, it is worth considering whether it is the innovation itself, or how it is being implemented, that will create problems.

The Amount of Flexibility in the New Way of Working

Andrew proposed that his staff and the patients who would be affected by the new protocol would need equivalent time and opportunities to adapt to it as other teams had had. The patients in question were familiar with the care of their lines, and were likely to have a view on any new way of managing them. Their views, as well as those of staff, would therefore influence whether the protocol could be successfully adopted (Grol and Grimashaw 2003, Scott et al. 2003, van Bokhoven et al. 2003).

Change can be introduced by: a pilot scheme that allows the new way of working to be tested in a small area, and reviewed before being rolled out more widely; running parallel programmes in which the new way of working is phased in whilst the old way is phased out; or by introducing the new way of working in its full form, and discontinuing the old way of working at once (sometimes described as a 'big bang' approach). The first two approaches have the advantage of not requiring everyone to change everything at once, but mean that the point at which the new way of working becomes the established norm takes longer to achieve. The big bang approach has the advantage of rapidity and clarity over the establishment of the new way of working, but may create negative feelings amongst those who find the change threatening (Golden 2006, Paton and McCalman 2008: 119–120, Pare et al. 2011). Andrew felt that although the new protocol had been piloted, because they had not been aware of, or involved in, this, his team would see it as being introduced using a big bang approach. His suggestion was that the members of his team who worked most often with the patients with long-term intravenous catheters should have the chance to visit the team who had piloted the new protocol, hear about the process, see how it worked, and feed back to patients and colleagues. This might enable staff to develop confidence in how the protocol worked, and allay concerns about it. It would also mean that the pilot was more likely to be seen as 'real' or credible. Andrew proposed a timeline for arranging visits, staff and patients learning about the new protocol, and his team's adoption of the new proto-col. His intention was to avoid seeming to oppose in principle, or reject, the new way of working, but to make its adoption realistic and achievable for his staff. He acknowledged that this approach would take a little longer, but felt that it would enable adequate preparations to be made, skills gained, and confidence instilled, rather than the new protocol being a sudden change that created uncertainty, resentment and resistance (Golden 2006, Pare et al. 2011).

After some discussion, Andrew's proposal was accepted, and when he met with his team, he was able to outline why the change was being requested, and what would be required of them (Hodges 2008, McLean 2011). He was also able to present it as a change, which had been piloted, and with which they and the patients who were affected would have support in adopting. Although his team generally still felt that the new protocol was unnecessary, with the investigation, planning, and negotiating that Andrew had done, the general response was of good humoured resignation at having to change things because of 'someone else's problem', rather than anger about a sud-den, unsupported, and apparently arbitrary imposition from above. It did not move the change to being led by the practitioners concerned, or make it a part of what might be considered emancipatory or transformational prac-tice development from Andrew's team's perspective (Wilson and McCormack 2006). However, it did highlight that it was a practice-based issue that had created a need for change, reduced negative reactions to it, and improved the way in which the adoption of inevitable change was likely to proceed.

Working on the people, as well as practical, aspects of change can make a potentially unpopular, imposed, change less problematic.

If You Are Told that Change Is Required:

Identify who requires it.
Find out why it is required.
Assess whether the innovation itself will be acceptable to those affected by it.
Think about whether the way the change is being implemented will affect
    responses to it.
Consider what might make the innovation more acceptable.
Be prepared to negotiate.

The two scenarios presented so far in this chapter address change that is introduced because of necessity of some kind. In other situations, change is not linked to any problem in practice, or an imposed change, but is suggested because someone has a new idea, that might enhance practice, and wants to try it out.

Suggesting Change because of a New Idea

Rachel works on a six-bed coronary care unit (CCU). She recently attended a conference where she heard a presentation about a CCU that had developed a group support programme for post-myocardial infarction (MI) patients and their families. The presentation indicated that participants found the programme a useful and non-threatening forum in which to ask questions, share experiences, and gain support. Rachel's unit uses a healthy living post-MI leaflet, but, following the conference, she felt that a peer support programme, which included family members, might be a beneficial addition to the service they provided. However, there was no evidence that there was a problem with the way her unit currently provided follow-up, so before sharing her idea with her colleagues, she wanted to be sure about the evidence on which she was proposing this innovation (Plastow 2006).

The Evidence behind the Idea

A range of types of evidence can contribute to developing ideas about changing practice, including: research, audit, clinical evaluation, case reports, and expert opinion (Sackett et al. 1996, Aleem et al. 2009, Hahn 2009). However, not all evidence is good evidence, and different types of evidence are good for different things. Knowing the value of any type of evidence, and how suitable it is to inform you about the subject in question, is important when you are deciding whether or not to suggest altering the way things are done.

The presentation that Rachel had heard was described on the conference papers as a research report. Research is defined as a rigorous and systematic process of gathering and analysing information, resulting in new knowledge being generated (Burton 2004, Hewitt-Taylor 2011). What constitutes a rigorous and systematic approach to gathering and analysing information depends on what information is being sought: the best approach to finding out whether a new drug is safe for long-term cardiac support is very different from the best way of finding out how it feels to be recovering from an MI. However, in both cases, the difference between doing research and other ways of gathering and analysing information is that the processes followed in research should be systematic and rigorous, so that the findings and conclusions are as accurate as possible a representation of the subject in question.

Audit and clinical evaluation have many similarities to research (Wade 2005). The processes used in research, audit, and clinical evaluation all aim to gather and analyse information, and should all follow systematic and rigorous processes (Wade 2005). The distinction between the three is often described as being that research investigates what should be done, audit investigates whether or not what should be done is being done, and evaluation examines how useful or effective something is, or what standard it achieves (Wade 2005, National Patient Safety Agency and National Research Ethics Service 2009). Some forms of research involve testing new interventions, with a view to using them in the future, whereas audit and clinical evaluation only involve an intervention or interventions that are already in use, or would be in use regardless of the audit or evaluation activity (National Patient Safety Agency and Research Ethics Service 2009).

Despite these distinctions, when you are reading a report, research, audit, and clinical evaluation can look very similar: they all usually give a background to the work, explain what was done or was happening, how the quality or worth of this was investigated, what this was deemed to mean, and what is recommended because of it. The study Rachel was interested in was described as an action research study. Action research involves practitioners looking at their own practice, instigating something that might improve or develop practice, and using research techniques to evaluate the effects of this development (Ferrance 2000, Parkin 2009: 14–32). It has similarities to emancipatory practice development, as described in Chapter 1, in so far as an area for development is identified by practitioners, action is planned, followed by evaluation of and reflection on that action. Where necessary and appropriate, further refinement of the original plan, with ongoing evaluation and development continues this process (Parkin 2009: 28–29). The study in question clearly fit this category, as the support programme was developed by practitioners, in response to their own reflections on possible new ways of working, and comments from patients. Aspects of it were then evaluated using research techniques, refinements were made, and ongoing evaluations and developments planned. This process has links with both research and evaluation: the techniques of research are used, but these are interlinked with a real world innovation in practice being developed and evaluated (Parkin 2009: 29). The report stated that the study did not require the approval of a National Health Service (NHS) research ethics committee, because it was deemed to be an evaluation of an innovation in practice, and was approved by the local governance group. Rachel was not completely clear about whether the study was really a research or an evaluation. For some purposes, including for decision-making about which route of approval is needed for a study, the distinction between research, audit, and clinical evaluation is important (National Patient Safety Agency and National Research Ethics Service 2009). However, if you want to use existing evidence to inform your practice, perhaps what matters most is not whether the study in question should be categorised as research, audit, or evaluation, but its quality, and whether or not it applies to your area of practice. For Rachel's purposes, whether the work she was reading should be labelled as research, action research, or evaluation was less important than whether the information presented was derived from a systematic and rigorous investigation of the pros and cons of this way of working, and gave an accurate picture of the benefits and challenges of setting up and facilitating this type of support group.

> *When you are deciding whether or not to use a piece of evidence to inform practice, a key issue is how systematically and rigorously that evidence was gathered.*

Other forms of evidence, which are usually much easier to distinguish from research, are case reports and expert opinion. Case reports usually report a case or cases of a particular condition, disorder, disease, or situation detail what happened in that case, analyse this, suggest and debate alternative explanations for it, and what this may mean for other situations. However, they do not generally adopt as systematic, detailed, or rigorous a process as research (Gopikrishna 2010). Expert opinion is exactly what it says it is: the opinion of an expert or experts in a particular field of work. Whilst this can be a valuable source of information, the basis for claims to expertise varies, and thus the value of expert opinion is variable. Expert opinion is not usually considered to be as strong a form of evidence as research, because the views of experts may not be the result of the systematic approach to enquiry, which is demanded in research (Gopikrishna 2010). Consensus expert view is generally seen as preferable to an individual's view, because it is less likely to be subjective. Often case reports and expert opinion are combined, as an expert in the field will provide a case report, in which they use their expertise to analyse the key issues involved in that case.

To help people to make decisions about what type of evidence they should pay most attention to, evidence was traditionally organised into hierarchies, with research described as the highest form of evidence (National Institute for Health and Clinical Excellence (NICE) 2005). One of the advantages of doing this was that it clarified that some forms of evidence are, in principle, more trustworthy than others. For example, research that is systematically conducted is generally a more reliable, or trustworthy, source of evidence than a report of a single case. However, using one hierarchy as the sole guide for the quality of all evidence misses the point that the quality of evidence is in part dependent on what it is being used for.

Types of Written Evidence that Might Inform Changes in Practice

Research
Evaluation
Audit
Case reports
Expert opinion

In hierarchies of evidence, quantitative research (sometimes also referred to as positivist research) is generally placed at the top of the hierarchy. Quantitative research, as the name suggests, quantifies things and sees truth as objective, not dependent on context or interpretation (McGrath and Johnson 2003, Lee 2006). The belief underpinning quantitative research is that, by using numbers, whether something works or not can be seen, and how likely it is that this should apply, equally, to most people within a certain population or group (referred to as generalisability) can be predicted (Lee 2006). A hierarchy in which quantitative research is always at the top can be problematic because, although good quality quantitative research may be the most safely generalisable evidence, some things cannot be effectively investigated that way, or generalised (Glasziou et al. 2004, NICE 2005).

The study that Rachel was interested in used qualitative methodology. Qualitative research, also sometimes referred to as 'naturalistic' or 'interpretivist' research, engages with words rather than numbers, and does not aim to find an answer that can be confidently applied to everyone in a given population (so generalisability is not its aim) (Kearney 2005, Goodman 2008). It looks at the meaning of human experiences and acknowledges that 'truth' may be subjective and interpreted differently by different people or in different circumstances (LoBindo-Wood and Haber 2005). Qualitative research is often used to enhance understanding of individual and subjective things such as feelings, values, or beliefs, and it therefore seemed an appropriate way to explore, in some depth, the experiences and views of people who had participated in support groups. Quantitative enquiry would have been useful for a study, which compared the clinical outcomes for patients who had different follow-ups; but for this study, qualitative methodology was very appropriate, and probably more useful than quantitative enquiry, although in many hierarchies it appears lower down the list.

Quantitative research
Quantifies things. Sees truth as objective. Seeks generalisability of findings.

Qualitative research
Engages with words. Sees truth as subjective. Seeks in-depth, personal insights. Does not aim to achieve generalisability.

Another problem with relying on hierarchies of evidence is that they deal with the type, not the quality, of evidence. Using a purely hierarchical approach might suggest that a poorly performed quantitative study was better than a very carefully constructed case report. Whilst in principle research should be a better form of evidence than a case report, a poorly conducted piece of research, which gives misleading results, is not good evidence. People will often say: 'research has shown that...' the question though is really: 'Has good quality research shown that...?'

For these reasons, there is now a move away from focusing purely on pre-specified hierarchies of evidence, to concentrating on how good individual pieces of evidence are, and how appropriate they are for the subject and situation in question (NICE 2005). So, as well as deciding on whether the study she had heard about was an appropriate type of evidence to use, Rachel also needed to evaluate its quality.

In decisions about whether or not to change practice, checking the quality of the evidence that exists is as important as deciding what type of evidence you have.

The Quality of the Evidence

Rachel had heard about the study she was interested in at a conference, but it is difficult to evaluate the quality of a study from a 20-minute presentation.

The conference abstract gave a reference to where the study had been published, so Rachel obtained the paper and evaluated this.

The right way to evaluate evidence depends on what type of evidence you have. The mainstay of evaluating any type of evidence though is to look at whether the way that the information was gathered is likely to mean that it is a true or accurate representation of reality, and whether there are any other possible explanations for what the evidence claims to show. Evaluation of some forms of evidence, and in particular research, should include certain considerations or steps, because there are particular things that should be included in research. Some general principles for evaluating research are shown in Figure 2.4, but exactly what you look for to determine the quality of a piece of research depends in part on the type of study it is. There are numerous frameworks and tools that can be used to guide you in evaluating different types of research, such as the CASP tools, which can be obtained at http://www.casp-uk.net/. The question you

---

What is the study about?

Study title/hypothesis/question/statement of intent

Study background

Does the literature review/background appear unbiased, and relevant to the study?

Study paradigm, design and methodology

Do the study paradigm, methodology, and design fit the subject?

Are the paradigm, design, and methodology congruent with each other?

Methods

Do these seem a reasonable approach to finding the information required?

Does the way the methods were used match the methodology/paradigm?

Does anything about the methods seem likely to produce misleading results?

Were any procedures or tools developed appropriately (piloted, discussed with experts)?

Sample

Was the sample and the way it was selected appropriate?

Would the way in which the sample was selected have placed any limitation on the results?

Was the response rate high enough (if relevant)?

Ethical issues

Were the ethical issues involved in the study considered? (This might include ethics review, informed consent, coercion to participate, potential harm, confidentiality, and anonymity.)

Data analysis

Was the right approach to data analysis used? (qualitative analysis for qualitative data) Were appropriate specific analysis procedures used? (which statistical tests were used and were these appropriate)

Figure 2.4 Principles of evaluating research

Reliability and validity/trustworthiness

Does it appear that the study was conducted systematically?

Was anything obvious missing?

Was there anything that might have meant that the results could be misleading, or due to something other than what was being investigated?

For quantitative research:

Were reliability, internal validity in terms of construct validity, content validity, criterion validity (where appropriate), and external validity addressed?

Were all the data accounted for (no missing results)

For qualitative research:

Are the steps the researcher took to ensure the 'truth' of their findings clear?

For mixed methods research:

Were the data analysis processes appropriate for the type of data in question, and was there evidence of appropriate integration of results?

Results/findings?

Are these clearly related to the study title/hypothesis/question/statement of intent?

Are they consistent with the methodology, methods, and sampling?

Are any other things which might have influenced the results accounted for?

Conclusions and recommendations

Do the conclusions and recommendations match the findings?

Are the conclusions presented with the appropriate degree of certainty given the methodology, methods, and findings?

Figure 2.4   (Continued)

are ultimately asking when you evaluate research is: was this a good way to try to find out about this subject, and was the study conducted rigorously and systematically, using the principles of the type of enquiry in question?

The study that Rachel was evaluating used qualitative methodology. She therefore looked at tools that can be used to evaluate qualitative research, and selected the appropriate CASP tool (http://www.casp-uk.net/wp content/uploads/2011/11/CASP_Qualitative_Appraisal_Checklist_14oct10.pdf). Figure 2.5 shows how Rachel evaluated the report. If the study had been quantitative, she would have used a different tool, such as the CASP tool for randomised controlled trials, or case control studies.

When the evidence that you have comes from case reports or expert opinion, evaluating it can be more difficult, because less clear-cut guidance exists about what should be included. However, a good rule of thumb when evaluating any evidence is: is the argument that is presented well-reasoned, logical, and systematic, and have all the possible reasons for cause and effect in the case in question been considered?

Was there a clear statement of aims? Yes. The study aimed to explore the experiences and views of people who used a post-MI peer and family support group. The objectives were to ascertain: the views of patients, the views of family members, what aspects of the group were useful to them, and what aspects of the group they did not find useful.

Was qualitative methodology appropriate? Yes, because the study looked in depth at people's individual experiences and views, and tried to understand their unique situations.

Study design: Group interviews, with semi-structured schedules. This method was appropriate for what the study sought to achieve. The report highlighted the pros and cons of using group rather than individual interviews, and why group interviews were chosen. The reason for the number and identity of participants in each group was discussed. There was no indication of whether any group members were dominant or non-participative: the assumption was that the groups worked. The discussions lasted between 60 and 90 minutes, suggesting some depth of discussion.

Was the recruitment strategy appropriate? Yes. All those who had participated in the support groups were invited to participate in the study. Anyone who did not respond was sent one follow-up invitation, in case the first was mislaid, but further follow-up was perceived to have the potential to be seen coercion to participate. The sample was small, which is usually appropriate in qualitative research as depth of enquiry needs to be achieved.

Were data collected in a way that addressed the research issue? Yes. The setting was a seminar room where the support groups had taken place, to create a familiar territory. The semi-structured schedule was provided, and seemed likely to address the research issues. The interviews were taped and transcribed to enhance data recall. Data saturation was not discussed, but the intention was to use this as the first cycle of action research, giving the option for follow-up on this cycle if more information was needed.

Was the relationship between the researcher and participants adequately considered? Yes. The study acknowledged that as the participants had been patients, or relatives of patients, on the CCU, and participated in the support groups, they might feel obliged to give favourable evaluations of the initiative. Attempts were made to minimise this by asking participants to share areas, which could be improved as well as positive aspects of provision, and encouraging them to develop on any comments that suggested the possibility of improvements.

Were ethical issues been taken into consideration? Yes. The study was approved through local governance processes, and was not deemed by the NHS Trust concerned to require Research Ethics Committee approval. Participants were given an explanation of what participation would entail, and that they could withdraw from the discussions at any time, without any consequence to their treatment or continued participation in support groups. As data were collected by face-to-face interactions, complete anonymity could not be promised, but data were anonymised. Participants were advised that the researcher would maintain confidentiality over information that was shared, and the group were asked to keep any information shared within the group confidential.

There was a potential for participants to feel intimidated by the group, or distressed by the things they discussed. However, this risk was felt to be minimised by participants having become used to participating in support groups, and by the research team being familiar with facilitating such groups.

Was the data analysis sufficiently rigorous? Yes. Data were analysed using thematic analysis. The themes were developed inductively, using ideas generated from the data, not predetermined codes. The themes identified were listed.

Figure 2.5 Evaluation using a CASP tool

(available at http://www.casp-uk.net/wpcontent/uploads/2011/11/CASP_Qualitative_ Appraisal_Checklist_14oct10.pdf) With kind permission of Critical Appraisal Skills Programme (CASP) www.casp-uk.net

The main points raised were noted as the group discussion progressed and informal feedback given to the participants to check that the researcher's interpretation of what was said was accurate. The findings included what people had found helpful, useful, or beneficial, and what had been problematic, and seemed to present unusual or 'one-off' experiences as well as the majority view. The study gave enough detail of the context it was carried out in to enable others to see whether the findings were likely to be transferable.

Was there a clear statement of findings?

The findings were clearly presented and matched the conclusions and recommendations made. The paper did not suggest that the findings were generalisable, which is usually the case in qualitative research. The study stated that it used the principles of Lincoln and Guba's (1985) criteria for qualitative research as quality indicators. Using these criteria, the study provided enough evidence of confirmability, bearing in mind the word limits of a journal article.

How valuable is the research?

The study provided information that Rachel thought would be useful for her own work. It identified that peer and family support groups could be valuable for patients and families after MI. It also provided some indication of what worked and what did not. It gave enough information about the study context for Rachel to think about what might or might not be transferable to her unit. Although it had limitations, it appeared to present an accurate picture of what was studied, and would be useful for Rachel in designing a group on her own unit.

Figure 2.5   (Continued)

Fitting All the Evidence Together

When you have one paper that seems to be good quality, relevant, evidence, it is tempting to think that this is reason enough to recommend a change in practice. However, it is always advisable to see if there is any more evidence that supports or contradicts it. If you have gathered all (or as much as is possible) of the available evidence, you will have a better idea of whether your idea really is worth trying, a greater chance of having a logical and reasoned argument for suggesting it, and less chance of encountering unexpected counterclaims to your suggestion when you present your case.

Having evaluated the paper that gave her the idea of setting up a peer and family support group, Rachel carried out a search to see what other evidence was available on this subject. The study she had did not address anything except the views of support group participants, and she thought that information about outcomes or measurable health parameters might be more convincing for some audiences. From her search, there appeared to be no other research about post-MI peer and family support groups. However, she did find some related articles. One was a small study that compared the outcomes for patients who attended a peer (but not family) support group after MI compared to those who had only had written information. It looked at lifestyle changes being adopted and adhered to, and reported compliance with drug therapy, and attendance at appointments. All were improved in those who attended the peer support groups. Rachel also found a qualitative study evaluating the effect of having families as well as peers involved in a support group, although this study focused on people who had type 2 diabetes. The study measured compliance with prescribed medications, and blood sugar control (which it reported were improved in patients who attended the family and peer support group). A third paper that she located reported on a qualitative exploration of people's experience of long-term neurological illness and how this was affected by attending a peer and family support group (it suggested that peer and family support groups were useful in improving some aspects of living with a long-term condition). These latter two studies both concerned different client group from Rachel's, but some of the principles, for example, those related to lifestyle adaptation, had similarities for her group, so she considered them worth adding to her sum of evidence. Rachel's search also provided her with two opinion pieces about the value of family and peer support for people who had heart disease, both suggesting that this was beneficial. This range of evidence enabled her to build up her picture of why, and on what basis, she thought that introducing a peer and family support group would be useful, and to have some certainty that there was no contradictory evidence. She was, however, aware that if her unit set up such a group it would be based on limited, if feasible, evidence.

However good a piece of evidence is, it will only be useful if it is relevant. An important part of deciding whether or not existing evidence should direct a change in practice is therefore to decide whether it is applicable to your area of practice. The presentation that Rachel had heard was given by nurses from a coronary care unit that was a regional centre, and much larger than hers. This might mean that the unit had more resources to devote to the development of a group, and a larger bank of potential participants, which would make it more viable. Conversely, it might be easier for patients from Rachel's unit to attend meetings, as they might have to travel less distance. Rachel also thought about what aspects of the studies that concerned people with type two diabetes and long-term neurological conditions might be transferable. The study about people with type two diabetes, for example, whilst conducted with a different client group, had some transferability as it dealt with similar issues in terms of taking medication, changing diet, and exercise habits.

Having evaluated the study that originally gave her the idea of introducing peer and family support groups, and looked for additional evidence, Rachel's next step was to float her idea with her colleagues, to see what their views were. Although she was enthusiastic about it, she would need to create interest and motivation in her colleagues in order to trial it.

Before making a recommendation for change: search for all the evidence, for and against your idea, evaluate its quality, and its applicability to your area of practice.

Summary

Changes in practice may be initiated, or required, for a variety of reasons, which will affect the steps that need to be taken to define, design, and plan for a new way of working. How the need for change is identified, and the idea of a new way of working introduced to those who will be required to do it is very important in terms of the likelihood of change being successful, and enduring long term. Not all change will be initiated by practitioners, based on their perceptions of what is needed. However, involving those who will need to work in a new way in its design, and planning change in a way that motivates them, and seeks to reduce the factors that might create opposition to change, is an important part of managing any type of change. Chapter 3 will, therefore, explore some of the issues involved in creating motivation for change.

Key Points

The best way to introduce an idea for change depends on why the innovation is being suggested.

Where a problem in practice exists, identifying exactly what the problem is, and its cause, enables innovation to address the cause, rather than the effect, of the issue.

Where change is imposed on a team, finding ways to maximise choice and control for those concerned can positively influence their acceptance of change.

It is important to fully evaluate all the available evidence related to a proposed innovation.

CASE STUDY

Joe works on a children's ward, where he noticed that paracetamol was often given to treat mild fever, although the general recommendation is that paracetamol should not be given solely for this purpose. He wanted to explore why people continued to use this approach.

How Did Joe Know that There Was a Problem, and What the Problem Was?

Joe thought that staff often handed over that they have given paracetamol to children who had mild fever, and that he frequently saw this written in the children's notes. However, in order to determine if this really was a problem, and what the problem was, he noted when this was mentioned at handover and checked the notes of children who were on the ward over a one-month period, to see how many really did receive paracetamol for what seemed to be mild fever alone. When he identified a case in point, he tried to find out, either by talking to the nurse concerned, or reading the notes, whether the paracetamol was actually given to treat mild fever, or whether it was given for another reason, such as the child also being in pain, or uncomfortable. He looked to see if there were any particular times when paracetamol was given to manage mild fever, or whether there was a particular group of children with whom this occurred. By carrying out this check, he was able to identify whether paracetamol really was very often given solely to treat mild fever, and, if so, when this seemed to happen.

How Did Joe Identify the Cause or Causes of the Problem?

Joe found that there was a consistent tendency for children to receive paracetamol to treat mild fever, but that this did not happen at any particular time, or with any particular group of children. His initial investigation also suggested that there were a number of causes for this, few of which were directly linked to the child's fever. He used the Seven S model to try to identify the underlying cause, or causes, of the problem.

Systems: There was no protocol available to guide staff about thresholds for administering paracetamol for fever.

Staff: Staff did not generally want to give paracetamol unnecessarily, but their level of experience and expertise varied, as did their confidence in discussing paracetamol administration with parents (some of whom were averse to the idea of not giving paracetamol to treat mild fever).

Staffing levels were generally thought to be fairly stretched, which meant that having lengthy discussions about paracetamol administration with parents was not always possible, and some staff took the path of least resistance when faced with a child who they did not really feel merited paracetamol administration, but whose parent was insistent on this course of action.

Shared beliefs/values: Whilst the ward had a shared 'unofficial' belief that ideally paracetamol should not be given unnecessarily, what was meant by 'unnecessary' varied between staff members, and parents also had differing views on this matter. Whilst there was a general acceptance that paracetamol should not be given to treat low-grade fever, parental requests and concern about increasing fever meant that there was no one agreed approach to when and why to administer paracetamol in relation to mild fever.

Strategy: There was no specific ward-based strategy for managing mild fever, or for teaching staff about paracetamol administration.

Structure: The care of the children on the ward was allocated to staff who were registered nurses and healthcare assistants. The registered nurses administered the medications, but where a healthcare assistant was caring for a child, they often requested paracetamol for a child, and were influential in whether or not the child received this.

Style of management: The ward was generally very democratically run, with everyone's opinion seen as valued. The ward manager did not adopt a hierarchical system of management.

Skills: The skill level of staff varied. Some of the registered nurses were newly qualified, whilst others had many years of experience. Similarly the healthcare assistants had differing levels of experience and training.

From the Analysis, How Did Joe Identify What Could Be Done to Address the Problem?

From his analysis, Joe felt that the core issues were that there was not clear guidance for ward staff on when paracetamol should or should not be given in association with mild fever. This not only meant that when staff were confronted with a child who had mild fever they were sometimes themselves unsure of whether or not to administer paracetamol, but found it hard to debate this point with any parents who were insistent on paracetamol being given.

Joe felt that whilst the democratic approach to management on the ward had many advantages, it did mean that sometimes there was a lack of uniformity of approach in key areas, which could be problematic. Having a guideline about the administration of paracetamol for mild fever might therefore, he felt, be useful, so that there was a clear baseline expectation, within which individuals could exercise their professional judgment in individual cases.

GUIDED WORK

This section revisits the learning outcomes covered in the chapter. You may want to complete it alone, or with colleagues.

1. Use appropriate approaches to identify and analyse problems in practice.

Think about a problem that exists in your workplace.

- Consider how you know that this is a problem, exactly what the problem is, when and where it happens, and what is its extent.
- Carry out a problem analysis to help you to identify the cause or causes of the problem (think about using approaches such as the Five Whys, Problem Tree analysis, Seven S model, or fishbone diagram).
- From the analysis, identify what could be done to address the problem.

2. Consider how control and choice for those affected by change can be maximised even in imposed change.

Think about a change that your workplace has been required to make, recently or in the past, and identify:

- Who required this?
- Why was it required?
- Was the innovation itself acceptable to the team concerned?
- Did the way people were told about the innovation influence their acceptance of it?
- Did the way the change was implemented affect responses to it?
- Was there anything else that particularly influenced (positively or negatively) acceptance of the innovation?
- Could anything have been done to make this change more acceptable?

3. Identify various types of evidence that might inform change and their relative value.

Identify an innovation that you would be interested in making in practice.

- Consider what type of evidence would be most useful to guide your decision-making about whether or not to attempt this innovation (for example, quantitative research, qualitative research, audit, and expert opinion).
- Carry out a search and see what information is available on this subject.
- List the types of evidence have you found, and how many pieces of each type of evidence there are.

- How useful do you think this range of evidence would be in enabling you to make decisions?

4. Understand the principles of evaluating evidence for use in practice.

- Select one of the pieces of evidence that you found in 3.
- Using an appropriate tool (one from this chapter or one of your own choosing) evaluate this evidence.
- List its key strengths.
- List its weaknesses.
- What weight would you give this evidence for the purposes of recommending a change in practice?

Additional Resources

Five Whys analysis:
http://www.isixsigma.com/tools-templates/cause-effect/determine-root-cause-5-whys/ and http://www.institute.nhs.uk/creativity_tools/creativity_tools/identifying_problems_-_root_cause_analysis_using5_whys.html

Fishbone diagram:
http://www.mycoted.com/Fishbone_Diagram and http://www.isixsigma.com/tools-templates/cause-effect/cause-and-effect-aka-fishbone-diagram/

Problem Tree analysis:
http://www.odi.org.uk/resources/details.asp?id=5258&title=problem-tree-analysis and http://www.iucn.org/about/work/programmes/forest/fp_our_work/fp_our_work_thematic/fp_our_work_flg/fp_forest_law_resources/fp_forest_law_resources_cna_tools/fp_forest_law_resources_cna_tools_3/

Seven S model:
http://www.valuebasedmanagement.net/methods_7S.html and http://www.c4eo.org.uk/changemodels/modeldescriptions/7smodel.aspx

Searching for evidence:
http://www.educationforhealth.org/data/files/resources/Literature-searching.pdf

Evaluating research:
http://www.medicine.ox.ac.uk/bandolier/painres/download/whatis/What_is_critical_appraisal.pdf http://www.casp-uk.net/

3
Motivation for Change

Chapter Learning Outcomes

After studying this chapter, the reader will be able to:

- Identify why the reason for a proposed change can affect its success
- Appreciate the elements of a proposed innovation that can affect enthusiasm for it
- Understand the value of making links between organisational or personal priorities and a proposed innovation
- Develop aims and objectives for change
- Plan change in a way that takes into account the influence of key players and opinion leaders.

Summary

The success of any innovation depends to a great extent on the enthusiasm of those who are required to do it. This chapter focuses on ways in which motivation for change can be established. It includes where and from whom the idea to change practice originates, what the change is, why it is being proposed, and what its likely advantages are. It discusses approaches to change management and how these may affect motivation; the value of having clear aims and objectives; how these can be developed; the importance of key players; and the effect of a fit between a proposed change and organisational and personal priorities.

Marissa is the ward manager of a 12-bed rehabilitation unit for people who have suffered spinal injuries. A range of professionals input into the rehabilitation programmes that the people on the unit undergo, including occupational therapists (OTs), physiotherapists, medical staff, and nurses.

Although it is a small, friendly, unit, communication about patients' rehabilitation programmes and discharge plans is not always easy to keep track of. Marissa recently began to be concerned about the number of occasions on which staff mentioned communication breakdowns to her. At around the same time, she received a letter of complaint and two incident reports that suggested patients had received inconsistent input, or contradictory advice, from different professionals.

Marissa felt that something needed to be done about communication, and that, as the ward manager, she was responsible for initiating this process.

Where Does Change Come from and Why?

Change is more likely to be successful if those who are required to do something differently see the reason for it as valid, and worth acting on (Ludwick and Doucette 2009, Pare et al. 2011). As the ward manager, Marissa felt that she had to take a lead role in addressing what appeared to be a problem with communication on the unit. She nonetheless wanted this to be seen as an issue experienced by the team, not one that primarily concerned her. She aimed to use a process that enabled the unit staff to own any problem that existed, see it as a valid concern, and develop their own solution to it (Palmer 2004, Pare et al. 2011). She also intended to use this as an opportunity to work towards a culture in which the staff reflected on their practice, thought about whether anything could be improved, and developed the habit of, and confidence in, trying new ways of working where appropriate. Using this approach might enable individuals, and the unit as a whole, to move in the direction of emancipatory practice development (Manley and McCormack 2003, Wilson and McCormack 2006), or transformational practice development (Dewing 2010, Walsh et al. 2011), as described in Chapter 1. To begin this process, Marissa invited all the staff who worked on the unit, from across disciplines, to a meeting to discuss the situation that had arisen. As she was aware that freeing the staff up to attend would be problematic, she also asked people who could not attend to send their views and ideas to her, so that she could share these with the group.

As Chapter 2 identified, for people to want to change the way they do things, they need to know why they should do so, what the benefits may be, and what will happen if they do not (Kotter 1995, Pare et al. 2011). Although Marissa aimed for the unit staff to devise and own any solution to the problem she was highlighting, she had to begin the process by explaining why she had called the meeting, what the benefits of thinking about the issue might be, and what could happen if nothing changed. When she did this, Marissa emphasised that although the complaint that had been received and incidents were important, it was the regular comments that she received from her colleagues rather than isolated incidents that were causing her concern. Her intention in adopting this stance was to present the problem as an issue that was affecting the staff themselves, and that it was in their interests to address. Her opening comments prompted some discussion, but the consensus was that communication did not always go as well as it might, and that practice in this area could beneficially be improved.

At this stage, Marissa felt that the reason for exploring different ways of working had been addressed, and those present, broadly speaking, agreed that there was a problem that needed to be resolved. In terms of what would happen if things did not change, Marissa wanted to avoid sounding as if she was issuing a threat, but she highlighted that it would probably be better to act before the situation became worse and further incidents occurred or complaints were made. She suggested that they should explore the problem together, and find a solution that they felt they could work with, rather than allowing things to deteriorate and being required to change their working habits in a way that they might not find acceptable. In this way, Marissa aimed to enable the staff to be proactive, understand, control, and own the way they decided to solve the problem. This was likely to increase the chance of any change in practice being successfully implemented (Paton and McCalman 2008: 29, Ludwick and Doucette 2009, Hall and Hord 2011: 148).

People are more likely to accept change if they can see why it is needed, and are involved in designing it.

Approaches to Change Management

Although Marissa did not ultimately want to lead the change process, at this stage she was acting as a change leader, highlighting a problem that people had reported to her and encouraging the team to find solutions to it. Scott et al. (2003) describe two types of change leadership: transactional leadership, in which compliance with change is achieved by providing material motivation and rewards, and transformational leadership, in which change is achieved because people are inspired to see things differently and thus perceive the need for change. Transformational leadership is clearly linked to transformational practice development, where practice develops as people reflect on, see a need for, and value in, altering the way they work (Dewing 2010, Walsh et al. 2011). Marissa's intention was to use a process, which would fall predominantly within the transformational approach to leading change, where the staff were enabled to identify a need for change, explore ideas about solutions to a problem, and empowered to select, implement, and evaluate these, rather than being told what they should do (Manley and McCormack 2003). However, there was also an implication that if the issue was not addressed, the situation might deteriorate, and a requirement to change working practice be imposed. This was closer to a transactional approach rather than a transformational one (Scott et al. 2003), and thus Marissa's approach did not fall completely within one model. Real-world change is a complex process, which is brought about by many competing needs, demands, and expectations, which often means that a single theory will not adequately address it. However, Marissa's main focus was strongly influenced by concepts such as transformational leadership (Scott et al. 2003) and emancipatory and transformational practice development (Manley and McCormack 2003, Wilson and McCormack 2006, Dewing 2010, Walsh et al. 2011). Her intention was to enable the staff to reflect on, own, and act on practice issues, rather than seeking solutions from outside, and, by so doing, to develop the skills, motivation, and confidence to continue to develop their practice.

Leadership and Change

Transactional leadership: compliance with change is achieved through material motivation and rewards.

Transformational leadership: people are inspired to see things differently and therefore perceive a need for change.

Chin and Benne (1985) identify three main approaches to motivating people to change their practice: the empirical rational, normative re-educative, and power coercive approaches. The empirical rational approach assumes that people will change the way things are done if they understand the reason for it, and it is in their own or the general best interests to do so. This approach focuses on explaining why a new way of doing things is being suggested, and presenting the evidence to support this. Although Marissa did not suggest a solution to the problem, there was an element of the empirical rational approach to the way she managed the situation: she explained why she was suggesting that there was a problem, and why the team might want to consider what could be done to address it.

Having a rationale for change is always important (McLean 2011), so nearly all change requires an element of the empirical rational approach. Nevertheless, however strong the rationale and evidence for this is, it is unlikely, on its own, to be enough to motivate people to change the way they work. Marissa could have designed an intervention to assist in communication, explained why it was needed, and why this approach should be used. However, as Chapters 4 and 5 will discuss, there are many reasons why people do not change their practice even when the evidence for doing so is strong. Marissa was aware of this, and wanted those who would be affected most by any new initiative to take the lead in designing it, so that it would be acceptable to them. In this respect, she focused more strongly on the normative re-educative than the empirical rational approach to managing change.

The normative re-educative approach focuses on the social and cultural implications of change, and explores why people may or may not favour a new way of working, even if it seems a logical idea, based on good evidence. This approach emphasises the implications of change for individuals and groups, based on their culture, beliefs, priorities, and values, and how this may influence their acceptance if change. It also considers it necessary for people to take an active part in, and own, change for it to happen. Working collaboratively with colleagues, seeking their ideas, and finding solutions, which will work for them, are key elements of this approach (Ludwick and Doucette 2009). This was the dominant ethos in Marissa's approach to change: exploring what staff's views and priorities were, and looking to engage those who would be required to participate in any change from the outset. The normative re-educative process focuses strongly on the people factors involved in change, and what, as Chapter 1 identified, Austin and Currie (2003) and McLean (2011) describe as the transition that they have to undergo to work in a new way. Using the normative re-educative process in whole or in part is usually essential to successfully change team practice because, as Chapter 1 identified, the outcome of any initiative is strongly influenced by how the people element of it is managed.

The power coercive approach to change is seen where political or economic power is used to achieve change: fear of the consequences of not doing things in the new way drive the change, not the value of the new way of working. This links with behavioural approaches to change management, where the focus is on persuading people to change their behaviour through positive or negative reinforcement, and contrasts with approaches that aim to create an understanding of why things could be done differently, or the intrinsic rewards of improving practice (Cameron and Green 2009: 19–24). A problem with this approach is that change may be implemented when you are looking but not otherwise, because no one believes in its value, except in order to stay out of trouble or to gain rewards. However, whilst this approach is often seen as unhelpful, some elements of it can be useful, and realistically necessary. Marissa wanted to avoid using a power coercive approach, but the triggers for the change that she was orchestrating included a complaint and two incident reports, which she felt it necessary to highlight as a part of the driver for change, because this was a reality that had to be worked with. In most cases, a mixture of the empirical rational, normative re-educative, and power coercive approaches are needed for effective change management, with each one brought into play appropriately for what you aim to achieve at the time, the nature of the team you are working with, and the reality of the situation.

Approaches to Change

Empirical rational: if people understand why change is needed, and can see the benefits of it, they will participate.

Normative re educative: the social and cultural implications of change are important factors in why people accept or do not accept innovation.

Power coercive: power, and fear of the consequences of not participating, is used to drive change.

Source: Chin and Benne (1985)

Managing change often requires a mix of approaches, depending on what needs to change, why change is needed, which individuals and teams need to participate, and what approach will work best with them.

What Needs to Be Done?

Marissa suggested to those at the meeting that they use a Problem Tree analysis (Hovland 2005) to try to identify what the causes of the problem were, and think about possible solutions. Various approaches to problem analysis are discussed in Chapter 1, and, as shown in Figure 3.1 using this approach enabled the group to identify the probable causes and consequences of the problem, to see links between causes, and to think about solutions. One of the issues, which was identified in the analysis was that because the team generally got on well, the assumption was that everyone would have the chance to pass messages on to each other, but that this assumption was flawed. The feeling was that whilst the unit's ethos of openness to different perspectives, collaboration, and mutual respect was valuable, it did not always result in effective communication about patient plans. Often, a patient had several different inputs in one day, and decisions about their

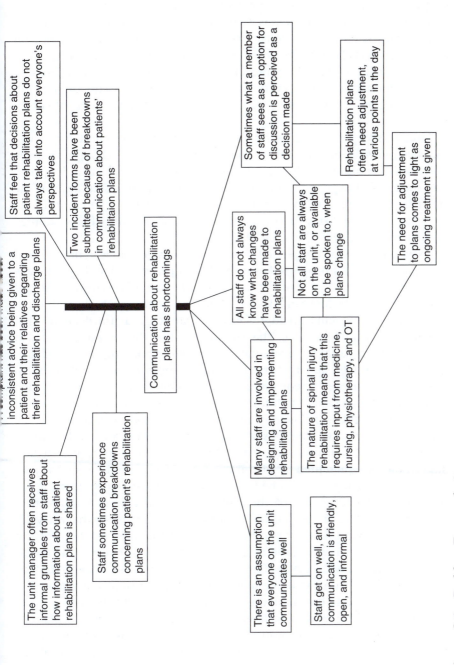

Figure 3.1 Problem Tree analysis

rehabilitation programme or discharge arrangements could therefore change frequently without everyone's input being considered together. A message from the problem analysis was that there was a need for more formal ongoing discussions about rehabilitation programmes with clear decision points, which each practitioner involved, and the patient concerned, knew about. To achieve this, the group decided that they should trial holding multidisciplinary meetings every Tuesday afternoon to discuss the rehabilitation programme and, where relevant, discharge plan, for each patient on the unit.

From this, those at the meeting knew why and by whom a need for change had been identified, what this would be, and why it was thought that the new way of working would assist in solving the problem. In addition, they had owned and explored the problem as a team, and the solution was the one that they had devised, not the one that was being imposed on them. These actions were likely to increase the likelihood of change being adopted (Welch and McCarville 2003, McLean 2011).

As well as knowing the general principles of what a change in practice will entail, it is useful for people to know the detail of exactly what they will have to do differently, and what the impact on them will be (Giangreco and Peccei 2005, Golden 2006, McLean 2011). Having decided that a weekly multidisciplinary meeting would be held, the group began to clarify the detail of what the meetings would look like. The decision was that they would be aimed at discussing each patient's rehabilitation program, including their discharge plan if appropriate, and that a representative from each discipline (nursing, OT, physiotherapy, medicine, and others as necessary), who had enough knowledge of each patient to inform the discussion, would attend. The meeting would be held every Tuesday afternoon from 14:00 to 16:00 hours. The nursing representative would usually be the person in charge of the unit or the members of staff who were caring for each group of patients. Medical staff would be represented by the middle grade doctor on duty, and physiotherapy and OT input would be by the OT or physiotherapist covering the unit, which would usually be the unit OT or physiotherapist, unless they were on leave. The timing was for Tuesday because it was felt that on Monday everyone was catching up on changes from the weekend, but if it was later, there might not be time to address key issues or referrals before the next weekend. Having devised this plan, everyone present knew the aim of the meetings, who should be represented at them, what was required of those attending, and how long the meetings were expected to last.

Although all those who were at the meeting knew what was planned and why, several staff had been unable to attend. It is always possible for there to be a discrepancy between what those introducing change think has been decided, and what those who are asked to do it perceive (Hall and

Hord 2011: 46). Messages may also be altered, misinterpreted, or distorted from the original as they filter through informal communication channels (Schifalacqua et al. 2009). In addition, change is more likely to be successful if those involved in and affected by it feel they are involved in the process, and communicated with (Jimmieson et al. 2008). Marissa therefore wrote notes from the meeting, emailed these to all staff, and put update notices in the communication book and staff room. Where individuals who had been unable to attend the meeting had provided input, she explained to them how their ideas had been presented and used in developing the proposed solution to the problem. This provided a reminder and clarification for those who had attended, and information for those who had not, so that exactly what was proposed, why this was proposed, and who had endorsed it was clear. Her message included the agreed aim of the project: To improve multi-disciplinary communication about inpatient rehabilitation programmes and discharge plans.

Change is likely to be less threatening if people know exactly what will be required of them.

Defining Aims and Objectives

Being clear about the aim of the proposed meetings was important, because it enabled people to decide whether it was something that they would be prepared to take the time to contribute towards achieving (Golden 2006). If the meetings were perceived as an event where general unit issues were discussed, people might make different decisions about prioritising attendance than if they knew that it had a more specific focus. Knowing the aim of a new way of working also makes it easier to stay focused, and to decide how much leeway there is for adjustments to the initial plan for change whilst still meeting its aim (Golden 2006). Clarifying that the aim of the proposed meetings was to improve communication about rehabilitation programmes meant that aspects of them could be tweaked, provided that members of the multidisciplinary team discussing and agreeing rehabilitation programmes remained their focus.

Having a clear aim also aids in planning the evaluation of change, because what should be evaluated is clear (van Bokhoven et al. 2003, Golden 2006). As the aim of the Spinal Unit's initiative was to improve multidisciplinary communication about rehabilitation programmes, the evaluation would ultimately be based around whether the meetings had improved communication between all the disciplines involved regarding rehabilitation programmes.

Within the aim of improving multidisciplinary communication about inpatient rehabilitation programmes and discharge plans, the group developed three specific objectives. These were

1. to hold weekly meetings between OTs, physiotherapists, nurses and medical staff;
2. to use these meetings to discuss and agree on the planned therapy, treatment and interventions required by all 12 inpatients on the unit;
3. to use the meetings to discuss patients' discharge plans (if relevant).

Having clear objectives within the main aim of a project is useful because it formally identifies exactly what will happen in order to achieve the aim. This particular development was relatively straightforward, but sometimes the apparent complexity of an innovation may detract from people adopting it (Hall and Hord 2011: 225). Breaking the larger vision of change down into clearly defined objectives can make it less threatening or overwhelming because it clarifies exactly what will have to be done. Equally, having objectives can avoid oversimplification, or unreasonable expectations about what can be achieved, by making explicit what will need to happen, and enabling those concerned to consider whether this really is achievable. These objectives made it clear that it was expected that multidisciplinary meetings would happen once a week, would be attended by OTs, physiotherapists, medical staff, and nurses, and that those attending would be expected to be able to discuss the rehabilitation, and possibly discharge, plans for the patients on the unit.

Clarifying what are and are not acceptable variations, any new way of working is important (Hall and Hord 2011: 50), and developing objectives can assist in this. The plan, which arose from the meeting that Marissa held, was to have meetings for two hours on a Tuesday. However, the objective was really to hold weekly meetings, and the detail of when this happened could change, provided this objective was met. If the meetings changed to every Wednesday morning, it would not matter, because the intention was to have focused meetings about rehabilitation programmes once a week, not to have meetings on a Tuesday afternoon. If, on the other hand, they changed to monthly, rather than weekly, meetings, it would matter, even if they were still on a Tuesday afternoon, as communication would not be frequent enough.

Objectives contribute to the evaluation of change as they clarify exactly what needs to be evaluated. Using the objectives as a guide, the evaluation of the meetings being proposed for the spinal injuries unit would include whether meetings happened every week, whether they focused on discussing rehabilitation programmes, and whether this improved communication related to these programmes. Other useful information might, as Chapter 9 will discuss, also come to light in the evaluation, for example, whether regular meetings enabled staff to better understand each other's perspectives. However, these core objectives would be the essential elements of the evaluation.

Exactly how objectives are stated partly depends on what you are doing, but one approach that is often described as useful is to use SMART objectives (Doran 1981). The SMART means that the objectives should be Specific, Measurable, Achievable, Relevant, and Time bound.

Having specific objectives means that exactly what you want to achieve should be very clear. Although the aim of the initiative Marissa was involved in was, 'To improve multidisciplinary communication about inpatient rehabilitation programmes', the objectives being specific gave a much clearer indication of what would be done in order to achieve this aim: weekly meetings with representatives from the key disciplines involved in patients' rehabilitation programmes would be held. Similarly, by stating that an objective of the meetings was to discuss inpatient rehabilitation programmes, the intended focus of the meetings was clear, and if people went off track could be noted.

SMART Objectives

Specific
Measurable
Achievable
Relevant
Time bound

Source: Doran (1981)

The measurable aspect of objectives may not always be possible, depending on what you are doing. It would be possible to measure the objective of holding meetings, by recording how many times meetings happened, how many were cancelled, how many times each discipline was able to attend, and how often plans were agreed at meetings. However, measurable objectives are only good for measurable things. Perhaps more important than measurable is that you should be able to decide whether or not you have achieved the objectives, using appropriate means.

The objectives of any new way of working should be achievable, or at least have the possibility of achievement. If you set objectives that would be ideal, but are completely impractical, the project will probably not succeed (Reed and Turner 2005, Cameron and Green 2009: 131). For the spinal unit's new initiative, daily meetings or multidisciplinary ward rounds were suggested as the ideal, but it was generally felt that, although this would give the best quality communication, it would not be achievable. Holding weekly meeting was considered to be achievable, and anything less frequent was thought to be unlikely to have the desired outcome. Weekly meetings were felt to represent a reasonable balance between the ideal and the achievable.

It might sound obvious that your objectives should be relevant to your aim, but the two can slide apart in the planning process. If the objectives for this innovation were purely about having multidisciplinary meetings, even if they happened, the aim of improving communication about rehabilitation programmes might not be met. By stating that one objective was to discuss inpatient rehabilitation programmes, the intention of the meetings was clearly focused on the aim of the initiative.

Having time-bound objectives can help you to think about whether your plans are realistic, and can enable you to keep your project on track (Clarke 2001). Marissa and her team aimed to introduce the weekly multidisciplinary meetings the next month, to pilot these for three months and then review them. Having a planned start date was important because, with the many competing demands on people's time, it would be easy for time to slip by and things to not happen. Equally, having a timetable can reduce the risk of rolling out a project before enough planning has been done or resources secured. Although this project did not require a great deal in terms of resources, it was felt that it would be useful to give people time to receive the information, and plan rotas and staff allocation to make Tuesday afternoon meetings viable. A project having a timeframe usually also makes it more manageable, because you can see what you should be doing at any given time, and whether things are on track or not. In addition, including a timeframe for evaluation can increase the acceptability of change, because it suggests that if things do not work out the innovation may be further modified or stopped, rather than being a fait accompli that will be continued regardless of its value.

Having sent out information, which stated the aims and objectives of the weekly meetings, Marissa's next step was to think about who might be able to take on key roles is refining, and rolling out, the new way of working.

Setting aims and objectives clarifies exactly what an innovation aims to achieve, and what practical steps will be required to achieve this.

Involving the Right People

Involving the right people in change is very important (Paton and McCalman 2008: 115). Marissa had taken the lead in identifying a problem and initiating the process of seeking a solution, but she did not want to manage the initiative, mainly because she felt that it was more likely to succeed if those who were involved in it on a day-to-day basis, took ownership of it (Paton and McCalman 2008: 29). She identified two main roles that were needed: a person to lead the whole project and process, and people to promote and oversee the new way of working within each discipline.

A key influence in the success of this initiative would be the person who took the lead role in managing it (Higgs and Rowland 2005, Golden 2006, Schulenkorf 2009). Marissa felt that, during the pilot phase of the project at least, a leadership, or change agent, role would be necessary, to make sure that the meetings happened, stayed on track, and became established. If not, although people agreed in principle that the meetings were important, and needed to remain focused, they might find other priorities or discussion points more pressing on the day. Golden (2006) suggests that those leading change need not only leadership qualities, but also expertise in the process being adopted. Marissa had identified that the unit's OT was not only a good leader, but also experienced in managing multidisciplinary meetings, which would be the key skill required. Change leaders or agents should also have personal conviction and motivation related to the change in question, and be able to explain why it is necessary (Bennett 2003, Golden 2006, Schulenkorf 2009). The idea of the meetings had come from the OT. She seemed very keen to see them happen and had been very clear in her explanation at the meeting about how this would assist in communication about rehabilitation plans. Good communication skills, openness to a broad range of perspectives, self-confidence and the ability to gain the trust of others are necessary attributes of change leaders or agents (Golden 2006, Schulenkorf 2009). The OT usually expressed her own views confidently, but Marissa had also noted that she was good at listening to others and their views. She was generally well thought of on the unit, and seemed to be someone whose views and requests would be respected. Marissa felt that she was the ideal choice to lead and facilitate the new way of working.

In addition to someone to lead the change, Marissa thought that it would be necessary to have a key representative from each discipline to either take responsibility for attending the meetings, or for nominating someone to attend. Multidisciplinary change management is discussed in more detail in Chapter 7, but these people would effectively be the change champions for their discipline. They would be those promoting the new way of working, and helping other people to adopt it, perhaps by encouraging the team they worked in to find ways of enabling someone to attend the meetings (Scott et al. 2003, Soo et al. 2009). In OT and physiotherapy, this was relatively straightforward, as one physiotherapist and one OT were primarily linked to the unit, and would usually be the people attending or delegating attendance. The OT would also, Marissa hoped, be the person leading the change. For nursing and medicine, one or two staff would be needed who could champion the new way of working. As one of the tasks, which would be likely to fall to them would be to encourage people to prioritise these meetings, and encourage them to attend, Marissa thought that self-confidence, and the respect of people in their team would be important for those undertaking this role (Golden 2006). It would also be important for them, like the change leader, to be enthusiastic about the project, and able to remind people of why it mattered (Bennett 2003, Schulenkorf 2010). Prioritising attendance amidst other demands could be a problem, and having someone who could understand and work with different perspectives, but still be assertive and enthusiastic in explaining why the meetings were important might be necessary (Golden 2006, Schulenkorf 2009). Marissa felt that the change leader and champions should also be clinically credible and respected so that they would be seen as understanding the conflicting demands of service provision (Golden 2006). This would better enable them to explore with staff how they could arrange workloads so that the right people could attend.

Planning change includes identifying people who have the skills, knowledge, and interests required to take on key roles in the process.

In addition to those who had an interest in, and skills that would be helpful to, this initiative, Marissa was aware of the importance of opinion leaders: people who were listened to, and whose opinion carried more weight than anyone else's (Iles and Cranfield 2004). Opinion leaders may not be high-profile people, but they have extra influence, for one reason or another (Hall and Hord 2011: 221). Because their views influence others, they can significantly help or hinder change (Iles and Cranfield 2004, Richens et al. 2004). When you are implementing change, you want them on your side if at all possible.

People may be opinion leaders because they are well respected and turned to when expert advice is needed (Hall and Hord 2011: 221). This was an additional reason for Marissa hoping that the OT would agree to lead the project: people generally respected her, her experience, and skills in managing difficult situations. She was often involved in multidisciplinary discharge planning and Marissa had noticed that her view was often sought, even if the matter in discussion was not especially related to her clinical specialty, because she was seen as having good judgment. She was also particularly respected by one of the neurologists who could be averse to new ideas, and her influence with him might be especially useful in securing medical staff attendance.

People may also be opinion leaders because they have the type of personality that everyone follows. They may not be such obvious choices to help you with your project, but involving them and having them onside is likely to be very useful. When the group was undertaking the problem analysis, Marissa noticed that one nurse tended to be negative about things that were suggested, and that this seemed to convince others that they would not work. She recalled that, in previous projects, when this person became negative about something, others also began to doubt. When the idea of meetings was suggested, this staff member immediately presented a problem of finding a day of the week that would be viable. Marissa therefore asked if she could suggest a good day. Tuesday afternoon was her idea, and by adopting it, others seemed to agree that this would be the best option. Marissa considered suggesting her for a championing role in ensuring someone could always attend from the nursing team, because this might mean that she felt committed to promoting, rather than detracting from, the initiative.

Key Influences on the Success of Change

Opinion leaders: those whose opinion counts, and will influence whether or not others accept change

Stakeholders: those who stand to gain or lose something because of change

Both groups hold influence over whether or not an innovation succeeds.

It is important to identify the major stakeholders in any change (Parkin 2009: 151, Schifalacqua et al. 2009), in addition to those whose opinion counts most. Stakeholders are those who stand to gain or lose something because of the new way of working. There were no individuals or groups who would obviously lose something because of the introduction of multidisciplinary meetings, because nothing was being stopped or removed. However, there is always the possibility of unknown or informal stakes being affected by change, such as how people have traditionally interacted, and the unofficial roles they have taken on or are seen by themselves or others as having (Carroll and Quijada 2004: ii17). Marissa was aware that some staff on the unit had informal communication roles, which they might feel were being lost. She knew, for example, that the physiotherapist and several of the junior doctors generally spoke at more length to one nurse than to anyone else, and that he often clarified to other staff what had been requested, and why. In the new scheme of things, although there was no reason why this could not continue, the value that was informally attached to his role might change. Marissa wondered whether it would be useful to ask him, as well as the other nurse, to be involved in championing the new way of working to nursing staff, emphasising that this was because he was already a key part of communication between disciplines.

It is useful to think about how much power each stakeholder has, and how much their desire to see change enacted or failing will influence others and the process as a whole (Parkin 2009: 151). This may be power that they wield because they have managerial power of veto: for example, the physiotherapist who was based on the unit would have power of veto if she decided not to be involved, as she could decline to attend and fail to send any colleague to attend on her behalf. Stakeholders may have no official power, but the possibly equal power of influence, which makes them an opinion leader as well as stakeholder. Marissa saw the nurse who she had noted was a key communicator between disciplines as an opinion leader as well as a key stakeholder because people liked him, and found him amusing. If he gently mocked an idea, other people would not take it seriously. On the other hand, if he promoted something, it had a good chance of happening, so his support was likely to be very important in making the project work.

> *Planning change includes identifying who will influence its success, and who they have influence over.*

Managerial Support

Whilst involving the right frontline staff in change is important, so too is gaining appropriate managerial support and involvement. Change is often described as coming from the 'bottom up' (initiated by frontline staff) or 'top down' (initiated and directed by management, and required of frontline staff) (Hall and Hord 2011: 12–15). Marissa intended to adopt a bottom-up approach in which frontline staff took the lead in designing and implementing change. However, she was also aware that managerial approval would be desirable, and possibly necessary.

Hall and Hord (2011: 12–15) suggest that although the top-down and bottom-up approaches to change are sometimes described as if only one can be selected, successful change usually requires a mix of both approaches. It is nearly always necessary for frontline staff to be on board for a new way of working to succeed, because they are usually the ones who have to do whatever it is that is required. However, there also usually needs to be an element of a top-down approach because managerial support for any change in practice is generally necessary (Allan 2007).

Although the initiative that Marissa was involved in primarily adopted a bottom-up approach, she discussed the plans that the team had developed with her manager, partly because if any issue arose regarding communication problems in the interim time, it would be known that the unit was already seeking to address the problem. She also wanted managerial support for the solution, and for her manager to understand why she was taking the approach she was (in terms of asking the unit staff to explore and agree a solution, and enabling them to lead the initiative).

Managerial support for new initiatives is usually needed in order to secure any necessary resources, and to achieve this, you may need to convince your manager that the initiative is important. The way in which you approach this may be different from how you try to convince colleagues of the value of a new way of working, because the issues that most concern them may be different. Budget holders generally have multiple demands on their resources and need to know that any costs, be they direct costs, time taken to change practice, or a risk of staff becoming disgruntled, will be balanced by the potential for positive outcomes. It is useful to be clear about the possible range of both short- and long-term benefits, which an innovation may bring, such as improved patient outcomes, patient satisfaction, increased efficiency, improved resource utilisation, staff satisfaction, or staff retention. Marissa explained that there were increasing concerns amongst staff on the unit about communication breakdowns leading to delays or inconsistencies in therapy, and that there had now been a complaint and two incident reports related to this. She emphasised that she wanted to act on this before it became a major issue. By being seen to be proactive in averting what could become a problem, she encouraged managerial buy in. She also gave an estimate of the likely cost and resourcing issues involved in the new initiative (Parkin 2009: 72). Although there were no direct costs, Marissa highlighted that the meetings happening was dependent on staffing levels being adequate to release people to attend. Other costs can include the cost of education or training, space, and equipment (Parkin 2009: 72). The change that Marissa was involved in did not require staff to undergo any additional training, or the purchase of equipment, but it did require a meeting venue. The unit had a meeting room, and the plan was to book this for Tuesday afternoons: having her manager's agreement for this meant that Marissa's room request was more likely to be honoured. This seemed a small thing, but Marissa knew that if a room could not be found, on a busy shift, people would soon go back to other work and abandon the meeting if they were 'wasting time' finding a room.

It is also generally useful to have a fairly clear, but flexible and negotiable, plan or idea of how you intend to orchestrate the proposed change, and the time span you are looking at, when you discuss it with your manager. If time and resources are being considered, showing that your plan is well thought out and viable is likely to make investing in it more attractive. It also makes it possible for the timing of any necessary resources to be considered, and any concurrent events or demands that might influence the proposed change to be brought to light. In Marissa's case, the intention was to commence the meetings in the next month, and as no real additional resources were needed, her manager simply needed to be aware that there would be a two-hour meeting, which staff would need to be free to attend and that the ward meeting room was booked for that time and purpose.

Managerial support may also be necessary in order to reduce any anxieties, which people have about possible adverse effects of change, such as complaints being made, or the legal implications of moving to a new way of working. Although this was not a major concern in Marissa's unit's case, it was useful to have managerial approval for the meetings in case questions were asked about why staff were using their time in this way. So, even in a predominantly bottom-up approach to change, managerial involvement and approval was vital.

You may find that your manager wants to be very involved in your project, and whilst this can be attractive because it ensures their buy in and may bring with it some authority, it is also worth considering the downsides of overt managerial involvement. It can be important from the point of view of keeping frontline colleagues on board that the project is clearly owned at workforce level and not seen as part of a management agenda. You may have to tread tactfully and carefully in winning support, making the right concessions and getting the right involvement from each level of staff without alienating others, or losing the focus of your project. Marissa's manager was pleased to hear about the meetings, and asked if Marissa wanted her to be involved. Marissa thanked her, and explained that she wanted the staff to feel it was their project, but that she would very much value the opportunity to come back and ask for her direct input if necessary. This retained her manager's buy in, as an expert adviser and overall manager, but avoided the meetings becoming a management requirement because of poor practice rather than a decision reached by frontline staff on how to develop and improve their practice.

Approaches to Change

Top down: initiated by management and required of frontline staff

Bottom up: initiated by frontline staff who convince management of the value of change

---

Top-down approaches to change are often seen as less likely to succeed than bottom-up approaches: but for change to be successful, it usually needs managerial support.

Taking into Account Organisational and Personal Priorities

A change in practice often has a better chance of success if it fits with or incorporates other things which are happening, which people see as important, or which they are required to do (McMurray et al. 2010). This applies both to acquiring managerial buy in for change, and securing the support of frontline staff. If you know that someone has a personal interest in something close to the proposed project, you may be able to use that to good effect. There is sometimes a fine line between someone's personal agenda fitting yours and you stepping on the toes of an idea they had, but trying to tie your work in with personal and organisational priorities is usually a good idea. Marissa considered whether there were any requirements of the unit, or people with interests or tasks to accomplish, which could be linked to the development of the multidisciplinary meetings. She knew that communication between disciplines was an organisational priority, and highlighted this link when speaking to her manager. She also knew that one of the junior doctors was required to undertake a project concerned with multidisciplinary working, so she planned to explore whether the proposed meetings could be incorporated as part of that project, perhaps not only with her acting as the change champion in medicine, but also working with others on the evaluation of the initiative.

Although it is useful to see whether or not you can tie in personal and organisational priorities to your project, it is also important to remember the core aim and objectives of your work, and to keep these central. This stops you moving too far away from what you originally planned, and makes it is less likely that, by taking on board or trying to incorporate other people's priorities, you will end up having agreed to take on a number of incompatible slants, which fragment, rather than complement and strengthen, the initiative.

> *Being clear about the aim of an innovation means that you can weigh up what other ideas or priorities you can incorporate without losing your focus.*

Summary

For any innovation to succeed, those who are required to do it have to see it as worthy of their attention and effort. Whether people see a new initiative in this way is influenced by where and from whom the idea originated, what exactly it involves, why it is being suggested, and what benefits it will bring. People's motivation to engage in new ways of working is also affected by how change is approached, how well the new way of working affects and is affected by organisational and personal priorities, and what other people think about the idea. How innovations in practice are developed and designed also influences whether they are likely to exist as solitary events, or be a part of the development of a culture of ongoing practice development for the individuals and teams involved.

These are all issues that it is useful to consider early on in developing plans for change, so that the new initiative has the best chance of success. Having considered them, the next step is to begin to plan the detail of exactly what needs to happen to bring about change. Chapter 4 will discuss planning change.

Key Points

Motivation for change is affected by what the suggested innovation is, where the idea came from, and its likely advantages.

Having clear aims and objectives helps to explain change, and keep it on track.

The way in which people are told about change often affects its success.

Key players and opinion leaders are important determinants of the success of change.

How far an innovation that matches personal and organisational priorities is likely to affect acceptance of it.

The success of any innovation depends on those who are required to work in a new way being prepared to participate.

CASE STUDY

Oliver is the Charge Nurse of a minor injuries unit. He has been asked by his manager to look into how the skills of the healthcare assistants (HCAs) on his unit could be developed to enable them to take on some of the roles currently undertaken by registered nurses (RNs), and to begin to change the way things are done in the department in order to make this happen.

Why Was the New Way of Working Proposed?

The changes Oliver was asked to make were a part of a review of what roles HCAs could develop in order to rationalise the staff required across the NHS Trust. It seemed unlikely to Oliver that the RNs on his team would find this an attractive reason to explore changing the way they worked, as it was likely to be seen a threat to their roles and employment. The advantage to the organisation did not seem likely to be as important to individuals as threats to their own jobs. The idea had been initiated by managerial staff, outside the clinical area, and had been precipitated largely by concerns over costs. Although there might be benefits for some HCAs in terms of role development, they would also be placed in a potentially problematic situation with their colleagues, who might perceive any gain for them as a threat. Developing this initiative as suggested seemed likely to create divisions and antagonism, rather than motivation for change.

How Was the Idea Developed and Change Approached?

The proposal was a top-down change. It appeared to rely largely on the empirical rational approach to change, with the provision of a reason (mainly cost, with some potential role development for HCAs) for the new way of working.

Did the Development Match any Priorities (Personal or Organisational) within the Team Concerned?

The development addressed organisational priorities, but would also afford HCAs who wanted to develop their roles in certain ways the opportunity to do so.

Who Played the Key Roles in Leading or Championing the New Way of Working?

The intention was for Oliver to take the lead role in determining how HCAs' roles could be developed, and in making changes within the department to enable this to happen.

Oliver felt that in order for this change in practice to succeed, it would need to be managed in a different way, with more focus on benefits to all those involved, and consideration of their priorities and views. At the same time, as this was a required activity, he had no choice but to find a way to meet the requirement to re-examine the roles of HCAs with a view to expanding their remit.

Oliver decided that the best way to approach this situation was to involve those most closely affected by the required change in planning a way forward. He called a meeting with his team, explained that the department was being asked to look at how roles could be expanded and adapted, and that he wanted everyone's input, so that they could design a proposal that would work for them, as well as the organisation. One of the staff asked if this was a way of getting HCAs to take on RN roles and making cost savings. Oliver admitted that this was probably a major driver for the suggestion, but that his opinion was that they should all think about how they would like to expand or develop their roles, so that any changes would enable, rather than threaten, them.

Why Was the New Way of Working Proposed?

The reason for the requirement to review HCAs' roles was unchanged by Oliver's actions, but the way he proposed to address it aimed to make the proposal as acceptable as possible to his team, and to create some role development for all staff.

Oliver felt that developing a clear aim for his team would be useful, because it would formalise their vision of what they were doing, and what they hoped to achieve.

The aim that the team developed was to explore how the skills of RNs and HCAs in the department could be developed in order to enhance and expand their roles.

The objectives they developed were

To identify the roles that RNs currently undertake
To identify the roles that HCAs currently undertake
To identify areas where there was overlap between the roles of HCAs and RNs
To identify areas in which HCAs could develop their roles
To identify areas in which RNs could develop their roles
To identify how these developments would enhance service provision

How Was the Idea Developed and Change Approached?

The proposed initiative would now have more input from frontline staff: the specific objectives had been designed and agreed by them, and now required managerial approval. Whilst the whole initiative was still a top-down change, imposed on staff, it had a greater element of a bottom-up approach than previously. The overall approach was therefore now a mix of the top-down and bottom-up approaches, which made it more likely to gain staff buy-in.

Rather than using an empirical rational approach as the dominant approach to managing change, there was now a stronger focus on the normative re-educative approach, taking into account people's concerns, and what mattered to them, which made any subsequent change in practice more likely to succeed. It also meant that staff had the opportunity to reflect on their current roles and remits, and to consider whether they wanted to develop these in a particular way.

Did the Development Match any Priorities (Personal or Organisational) within the Team Concerned?

By including the possibility of role development for both HCAs and RNs, and asking staff to be involved in identifying their roles and how these could be developed, rather than suggesting the focus would only be on HCAs expanding their role, Oliver intended to make the organisational goal fit, as far as it could, the personal aspirations or interests of as many staff as possible.

Who Played the Key Roles in Leading or Championing the New Way of Working?

The initial intention had been that the key role in this review would be played by Oliver, as the departmental manager. However, his intention was that the lead roles would be taken by an RN to collate the activities and views of RNs and an HCA to collate the activities and views of HCAs. These would then be discussed by the team, and plans for development and role realignment made from this. It would mean that those who were required to work in any new way were those most closely associated with developing the plan, and thus had a degree of involvement in and ownership of the decisions made. Oliver asked the team to consider who would want to take on lead roles for each group.

Oliver would still need to meet the managerial requirement to review roles, and there was a strong possibility that the recommendations he and his team made for change would need to be modified and a compromise sought between their goals and aspirations and those of the organisation as a whole. However, by using the approach he did, Oliver hoped that his own staff would gain as much as they could from the situation, and maintain as much choice, control, and personal and professional development as possible.

GUIDED WORK

This section revisits the learning outcomes covered in the chapter. You may want to complete it alone, or with colleagues.

1. Identify why the reason for a proposed change can affect its success.

Identify a change in practice that you have been involved in, or are aware of, and consider whether:

- Those involved knew why the new way of working was proposed.
- Those involved knew what the benefits of the innovation were thought to be.
- This affected the ease with which the innovation was implemented.

2. Appreciate the elements of a proposed innovation that can affect enthusiasm for it.

In relation to the change in practice listed above, identify:

- Whose idea it was?
- What the aim of the innovation was?
- Whether exactly what the innovation would involve was clear?
- How change was approached (for example, predominantly top down/bottom up, were the empirical rational, power coercive, or normative re-educative approaches used, in whole or in part).
- Who the major stakeholders were, and whether they supported or opposed the innovation.
- Who the opinion leaders were, and whether they supported or opposed the innovation.

Suggest how each of these factors might have affected the success of the innovation.

3. Understand the value of making links between organisational or personal priorities and a proposed innovation.

In relation to the change in practice listed above, identify whether:

- The innovation matched or conflicted with any of the priorities of the team or organisation concerned.
- The innovation matched or conflicted with the personal priorities of any individuals.

For both responses, consider what effect this might have had on the ease with which change was implemented.

4. Develop aims and objectives for change.

Identify a change in practice that you would be interested in making.

- State the aim of the innovation.
- List the objectives of this innovation (you may wish to use SMART to guide you).

5. Plan change in a way that takes into account the influence of key stakeholders and opinion leaders.

For the change in practice that you have identified in 4:

- List the key stakeholders who would be affected by this change.
- Think about whether they would be likely to support or oppose it, and why.
- Consider how you might reduce any opposition to and increase their support for this innovation.
- List those whose opinion would influence the success of this change.
- Identify why their opinion counts.
- Think about whether they would be likely to support or oppose it, and why.
- Consider how you might reduce any opposition to and increase their support for this innovation.

Additional Resources

Discussion of Chin and Benne's work:
http://www.sedl.org/change/facilitate/approaches.html

Additional Resources *continued*

Setting SMART objectives:
http://www.thepracticeofleadership.net/setting-smart-objectives

Key players:
http://www.change-management.com/tutorial-cm-basics-who-mod2.htm

Change agents:
http://www.themanager.org/strategy/change_agent.htm   and   http://www.isix
sigma.com/implementation/change-management-implementation/making-
good-change-agents-attitude-knowledge-skills/

4

Planning Change

Chapter Learning Outcomes

After studying this chapter, the reader will be able to:

- Identify driving and restraining forces that might affect the success of an innovation
- Understand how readiness for change at individual and team level influence its success
- Appreciate how different approaches to giving information about change may be successful with different audiences
- Develop a plan for change that includes human and practical elements
- Set a realistic timescale for introducing innovation.

Summary

This chapter focuses on planning change. It begins by discussing the need to assess the factors that are likely to drive or restrain change, including human factors, resources, and training needs. This is followed by a description of the process of assessing individual and corporate readiness for change, and an overview of some of the things that should be considered in giving information about change as well as setting timescales for change.

Leila works as part of a team of school nurses who cover ten primary schools. She is interested in encouraging healthy eating in children, and her opinion is that the best way to achieve this is to work with their parents. To this end, she has had the idea of having regular, but informal, drop-in sessions, at which parents can get information, advice and support about assisting their children to eat a healthy diet. Her proposed aim is to provide an opportunity for the parents of primary school children to access information, advice, and support related to healthy eating. Within this overall aim, the objectives of her proposed project are

- to hold weekly drop-in session for the parents of primary school children;
- to provide an opportunity for the parents of primary school children to discuss nutritional issues;
- to give parents a chance to suggest ways in which information sharing and support regarding healthy eating could be improved.

Leila included the last objective because she was aware that whilst she thought that this approach would be helpful, parents might have other ideas about what would work best for them, which the project would give them the opportunity to discuss.

Before telling the team she worked with about her idea, Leila discussed it with a colleague, to see if it seemed reasonable. Her colleague was enthusiastic, and wanted to be involved in the project. Leila then discussed the proposal with her manager, because, without her approval, the project would not be able to go ahead, however enthusiastic her colleagues were (Allan 2007). Nonetheless, whilst she needed managerial approval, Leila saw her idea as falling within the bottom-up, rather than top-down, approach to change (Hall and Hord 2011: 12). It was the idea of a frontline practitioner, who was not in a managerial position, or a particularly senior member of the team. Her manager liked her idea, but needed more specific information on how the project would work, resourcing, and costs, before she could endorse it.

In order to obtain managerial approval, and for her project to proceed from being a good idea to an achievable reality, Leila therefore needed to do some detailed planning, including the people, steps, and resources that would be needed, as well as the timescale over which the change would happen (Hall and Hord 2011: 149–150). Some of these things were obvious, but thinking every detail through meant that she was less likely to miss anything, and that she would have a good idea of how everything would fit together to achieve her aim. Having a clear plan would also allow Leila to give her colleagues enough detail about what exactly she was proposing to them to be able to decide whether they felt they could work with it or not.

Thinking about what is required or needs to be done for change to happen includes identifying the things that will assist in or hinder change from happening (Lewin 1951, Parkin 2009: 152–153). Identifying these enables you to plan how you can lessen the things that may stop change from happening, and add to the things that will drive it. Unless these issues are addressed at the planning stage, an excellent idea, whose execution stumbles frequently, or which never happens.

Driving and Restraining Forces

One of the things that Leila thought about when she was planning her initiative was what would help to take it forward, and what would stand in the way of it happening. Assessing these factors has been described as 'force field analysis' (Lewin 1951). The things, or forces, which are likely to positively affect change are described as driving forces, or facilitators of change (those that will help to drive forward or facilitate change), and those that will inhibit change as restraining forces (those that will act against or restrain it) (Lewin 1951, Parkin 2009: 152–153). For change to be successful, the overall driving force needs to outweigh the restraining force. The driving and restraining forces may be related to each other, or unrelated, but the overall strength needs to be positive to move change forward, and the stronger the positive force, theoretically at least, the less problematic implementing change will be. Figure 4.1 illustrates the forces that affect the success of change.

If the forces driving a change do not sufficiently outweigh the restraining forces, something needs to alter before an innovation can succeed. Ideally, you should aim to reduce the restraining forces and increase the driving ones. However, of the two actions, finding ways to reduce the restraining forces is usually the more vital, because if you increase the driving forces without addressing the restraining, or negative, forces, the tension between the two also increases (Iles and Cranfield 2004). If the negative forces are reduced, there is likely to be less resistance to the force of change, which creates a smoother pathway. As Leila considered the various aspects of her proposed project, and the practicalities of what would need to be done, she thought about how they could be achieved in a way that not only reduced the possible restraining forces, but also built upon, or added to, the driving forces.

If the forces that restrain change are greater than the forces driving it, an innovation will not succeed.

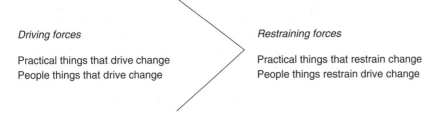

Driving forces

Practical things that drive change
People things that drive change

Restraining forces

Practical things that restrain change
People things restrain drive change

Figure 4.1   Successful change

When you are planning change, the processes that will be required, and the practicalities of what needs to happen to bring about a new way of working, are important. However, as Chapters 1 and 2 identified, even when the proposed change mainly deals with procedural or mechanistic alterations in workplace practice, there are usually significant people factors to consider (Paton and McCalman 2008: 21–25). As well as identifying and planning for the practical drivers and facilitators of change, it is therefore usually equally, and often more, necessary to consider the human factors that will drive or restrain change for individuals, groups, and organisations (Grol and Grimashaw 2003, Paton ad McCalman 2008: 21–25). Neglecting these can mean that however well resourced or technically sound the change you are proposing is, it fails because those who are required to do it do not do so. Chapter 5 discusses resistance to change in more detail, but thinking about the human factors involved in change, and what you can do to make your plans become more attractive, is an important part of planning change.

Leila identified that her project would need resources in terms of staff time, materials to distribute to parents, and a room at the school in question, but none of these were likely to create a significant restraining force if the people involved were enthusiastic about her idea. For her project to be successful, the most important driving and restraining forces rested with her colleagues, key school staff, and the parents of children at the schools in question. Because these were likely to be the key factors, Leila began her planning by thinking about the things that might affect people's enthusiasm for her project.

Developing Enthusiasm

Chapter 3 discussed things that can increase people's motivation for change, and these were amongst the issues that Leila considered in planning her initiative. A part of this was whether her plans would contribute to fulfilling the requirements or priorities of her organisation (McMurray et al. 2010). The team she worked with were required to demonstrate that they were doing something to promote healthy eating, and their ongoing remit included building on the health promotion work that they did in schools, particularly in relation to childhood obesity. Her idea would contribute towards achieving this. She also considered how far her plans might fit the priorities of schools concerned: the latest inspection report (OFSTED) for a school she aimed to approach about the project had recommended they develop their liaison and working with parents, which this project might feed into.

On a personal level, Leila had heard some of her colleagues commenting that as they now worked across several sites, having previously been based in one or across two schools, they did not have the opportunity to get to know staff in the schools very well. She wondered if having one or two members of staff involved with the project at each school would enable people to use it as an opportunity to get to know the staff and parents at a particular school a little better. That might, for some, be a driving force because it would mean that the initiative could be used to develop something that mattered to them (McMurray et al. 2010).

Another potential driving or restraining force that Leila identified within her own team was whether or not her colleagues considered it important to try to address healthy eating. Although this was an organisational requirement, if people were not convinced of its importance, they might still not see it as a priority, or be keen to participate. Alongside this, the priority which people saw this as holding would influence whether they felt they had the time to take on this way of working. Further driving or restraining forces might be people's views on whether this was a good way to promote healthy eating and whether they felt confident about working in this way. From the schools' point of view, the likely people centred driving forces were if head teachers or any individual teachers were particularly interested in initiatives aimed at promoting healthy eating, and how they felt about parents dropping in for sessions at the school. From the parents' perspective, the driving or restraining forces would include: whether or not they wanted to access information or support related to healthy eating; whether they were made aware of this initiative; whether the drop-in sessions looked interesting; and if they were facilitated in a manner that encouraged attendance.

Organisational priorities may not be a priority for individuals, and may not be enough to make people want to change the way they work.

Resources Needed

Although thinking about the people side of change is important, the material and practical aspects also matter. Resources can be a driving or restraining factor in change, because if they are readily available it will help to move change forward, but if they are not, it is likely to restrain change (Grol and Grimashaw 2003, Golden 2006). A vital part of planning change is therefore determining the resources that will be needed, and how they will be secured (Hall and Hord 2011: 149, MacPhee and Suryaparkash 2012). It is often impossible to get all the resources you would ideally like, so as well as thinking about what you need, prioritising what you must have, what you would find very useful, and what would be helpful but a luxury is sensible (Golden 2006). Knowing what you absolutely need is important because without this you cannot proceed. It can also be useful to think not only about what you could manage without, but also about what other people would be happy to manage without, and what the effect of this on the forces driving and restraining change might be. You might be happy to work with less than ideal resources, at least initially, but the extra workload or inconvenience might be a restraining force for others, which would tip the balance of the force driving change from positive to negative. If your project will last some time, it is also useful to try to break the resources you will need into stages, so that you have an idea of what will be needed at each point in time. Leila identified that she needed time (to devote to designing and setting up the project, liaising with school staff, writing letters, and then running the project day to day), the cost of the letters and posters that would be used to inform parents about the initiative, and a room at the school or schools involved.

The cost of the time required to facilitate a change project can be a key factor in its success (MacPhee and Suryaparkash 2012), and her time and her colleagues' time was the major cost that Leila's initiative would incur. She estimated that this would be one day a week for two months for planning and setting up the initial project, but once the initiative was underway it would be approximately three hours per week, per group running. She also identified that she would need time for the end of the project to evaluate it. Leila had been told that, in principle, if the plan she presented to her manager seemed reasonable she would be given the time for the project. However, she was aware that there was unlikely to be any reduction in other aspects of her or anyone else's workload to compensate for this project, so the reality was that it would be acceptable for her to use her time in this way, provided that she organised her other work to accommodate it. She was prepared to work with this, and at least initially stretch her hours a little, but was aware that for others, slotting an extra activity into a busy work schedule was likely to be a restraining force, especially if they were not fully convinced of the value of the project. This influenced how she planned to introduce the innovation: she thought it would be best to start by piloting it at one school, with herself and her colleague who had expressed enthusiasm for the project facilitating the group, rather than expecting others to reschedule their workload or devote additional hours to it. This would also allow the initiative to be tested, and reviewed, before wider implementation was attempted.

In addition to the resources she needed, Leila considered what other demands for them were likely to be competing with hers (Palmer 2004, Golden 2006). If numerous claims are already being made on limited resources, and your request is not seen as a priority, it may be better to wait, and develop a successful change in practice later, than to push ahead and fail (Palmer 2004). Leila knew that there were almost certain to be competing demands on rooms at most schools, and that having a room would be important because if she was searching for one on the day any parents who were trying to attend the session would probably lose interest and go home. In her own team, a number of new initiatives were apparently required, but none were, as far as she was aware, currently proposed or underway, so these should not be competing with hers for time or resources. This created an incentive for her to try to get her own project approved and underway before other ideas did begin to compete with it.

Determining whether a new way of working will require people to gain any additional skills or knowledge is a part of planning change (Golden 2006, NICE 2007, Hall and Hord 2011: 149). If it will, how these skills will be acquired (for example, through formal study, training sessions, or visits to other wards or departments), and whether they will need to be assessed should be considered (NICE 2007). It is also useful to think about whether any necessary training will be seen as a driving or restraining force, for example, an opportunity to acquire new and useful skills, or a drain on people's valuable time. Leila did not think that the other members of the team would need any new knowledge to participate in this project, as they routinely gave advice on healthy eating. Their knowledge would be supported by healthy eating leaflets, which were already available and with which they were familiar. If the pilot showed the initiative to be worth expanding, some staff, especially those with less experience, might need to gain confidence in facilitating this type of group. Leila thought that this could be most effectively achieved by them sharing group facilitation with a more experienced colleague until they felt comfortable to work alone, rather than through formal training. This would be one advantage of starting with a pilot of one or two groups, which other staff could participate in from time to time.

If training is needed, the sequence in which people access this merits some thought: people who are leading the change generally require early input, because they need to be knowledgeable about the new way of working from the outset. However, it is also worth considering the effect of the sequence of training on people's acceptance of change. Enabling someone who is not particularly enthusiastic about an innovation to access the first round of training may give them a role in helping others to develop the necessary skills, and bring them on board to support the change in practice. During the pilot, Leila planned not only to invite people to participate in the drop-in sessions on an ad hoc basis if they were interested in seeing how these ran, but also to ask for volunteers to provide cover for leave. Her intention was to use these approaches as an opportunity to help her colleagues to gain interest or confidence in facilitating the groups. She had in mind to particularly ask two people to help out: one who she suspected would oppose the plan but would perhaps come on board if she was involved, knowledge-able, and able to explain it to others; and one who was fairly newly qualified, and often appeared to be lacking in confidence, but who might then be keen to participate.

Having adequate resources for an innovation is important: without these, the effort required to make change happen is likely to become a restraining force.

Having considered the general driving and restraining forces that might affect her initiative, Leila considered how ready the individuals and groups who might be involved were for change.

Resource Considerations in Planning Change

Time
Materials
Equipment
Physical space
Training
Are these resources available?
Is anyone competing with you for them?

Assessing Readiness for Change

Readiness for change has been described as the extent to which individuals and groups are inclined not only to accept in principle, but also to adopt, a particular plan for change (Pare et al. 2011). It is usually seen as exist-ing on a continuum, from being ready to adapt to change (high readiness for change) to not being at all ready to undergo change (low readiness for change) (Holt et al. 2007, Pare et al. 2011). Readiness for change can also be seen in individual terms: how ready individuals are to adopt a new way of working, and organisational terms: how ready teams or organisations are to do this. The individual and organisational elements of readiness for change can also affect, and be affected by, one another.

Weiner et al. (2008) suggest that readiness for change includes struc-tural elements (such as the resources and systems that are needed), and psychological elements (people's attitudes, beliefs, and intentions). Other writers describe how readiness for change includes individual's cognitive and emotional acceptance of change: whether they think in theory it is a good idea (cognitive readiness) and whether it is something that they themselves feel able and willing to engage in (emotional readiness) (Pare et al. 2011). Sometimes these aspects of readiness for change are not easy to separate, and impact on one another. In structural terms, Leila would need a room at the school in order to meet with parents. However, the psychological elements of readiness for change would be likely to affect this in terms of the priority that was afforded to providing such a room. If the head teacher did not think that holding the group was a good idea because she did not see a need for it or understand the purpose of it (low cognitive readiness for change) or did not want school nurses intruding because she had previous negative experiences of such events (low emotional readiness for change) it might present as a structural issue of a room apparently not being available.

Things that affect resistance to change are discussed in more detail in Chapter 5, but assessment of individual and group readiness for change is an important part of planning any new way of working. The decision about when and how to initiate change will include how many people are ready for the change that is proposed, what weight of opinion, or driving force, they represent and whether this means you can go ahead with implementing change or not. Even if you have a very well-planned project, and have been promised resources and funding to achieve it, it will not be a success if no one actually does it.

Assessing Readiness for Change Includes Thinking about whether

People understand why change is being proposed.
People are convinced that change is needed.
People are willing, in principle, to change the way they work.
People feel able to work in the new way.
People actually intend to change the way they work.
The necessary resources are available.

Assessing readiness for change includes thinking not only about how ready people are to change, but also about how individuals will influence one another.

One way of assessing readiness for change is to use a model, or theory, to guide you as to whether or not people are ready for a new way of working. Not everyone will fit neatly into any stage of a model or theory, but using such a tool can help you to decide where you are at, and the tasks you have to achieve to get further on. Prochaska and Diclemante's (1992) model of readiness for change describes the stages of readiness as pre-contemplation, contemplation, determination to change, action, and maintenance of new practice. Although Prochaska and Diclemante's (1992) work is based on changing personal behaviour, not professional practice, it can still be a useful framework within which to consider one's own and colleagues' readiness for new practice.

Stages of Readiness for Change

Pre-contemplation
Contemplation
Determination to change
Action
Maintenance

Source: Prochaska and Diclemante (1992)

Pre-contemplation is the stage at which people are not contemplating, or willing to contemplate, change. They are either unaware of any suggestion that change should happen, or are aware of proposals for change but do not want it to happen. If the majority of the people who will need to change their practice are at this stage, something has to happen before things can move forward. Leila felt that, within the nursing team, there were relatively few people at this stage, as they were all aware that the team was required to show that they were working towards having a greater input on healthy eating. Whilst there were varying degrees of enthusiasm for doing this, there was a broad acceptance that someone would have to do something and that some new initiatives were inevitable. There were a couple of staff who simply saw this requirement as the latest fad, and thought that if they did nothing it would soon pass (Welch and McCarville 2003, Parkin 2009: 7), but by and large there was acceptance that at the very least something had to be seen to be done. By tying her project to this acknowledgement, Leila hoped to minimise the chances of team members being at the pre-contemplation stage. She was less sure of whether schools would see this as a necessary innovation. What was most likely was that there would be ambivalence to it: it would be seen as potentially useful, but not a priority. This might be most closely linked to Prochaska and Diclemante's (1992) next stage: contemplation.

At the contemplation stage, people have moved beyond dismissing the idea of change, and are thinking about it and weighing up its pros and cons. They have still not decided to change anything, but it is a possibility. Leila felt that some of her team, and many school staff, would be at this stage, where the idea was not rejected out of hand, but was not yet a convincing reality, or a priority to act on. She designed her approach on this premise, with the intention of building on the slight tendency towards readiness for change that most staff would probably have.

The next stage of Prochaska and Diclemante's model is preparation for change, or determination to change. At this point, the person or people concerned have decided that change is a good idea and are ready to participate. Leila thought that she and her colleague who was keen to work with her on the project were at this stage, and that there was at least one school where the head teacher would easily move from contemplation to preparation for change.

Ways of Introducing Change

Pilot
Parallel programmes
'Big bang'

Assessing whether the people who will need to be involved in any change you propose are ready for it is a key aspect of making a decision about whether or not to try to change practice at all, whether now is a good time to do it, and how, and at what pace, you should aim to bring about change. As Chapter 2 identified, change can be introduced via a pilot scheme, which allows the new way of working to be tested on a small area first, and reviewed before being rolled out more widely. Another option is to run parallel programmes, phasing a new way of working in whilst phasing the old way of working out. These both have the advantage of not requiring everyone to change everything at once, but mean that the full form of the new way of working takes longer to arrive. A third approach is to introduce the new way of working in its full form, and discontinue the old way of working at once (the 'big bang' approach). This means that the new approach is introduced promptly, and across the organisation as a whole, but may create negative feelings amongst those who find it threatening (Golden 2006, Paton and McCalman 2008: 119–120, Pare et al. 2011). Leila felt that at this stage she had enough people who were ready for change to implement her idea in one school, as a pilot. By introducing the project in this way, she thought that other staff, who were still at the pre-contemplation or contemplation stage, could see how things worked and the results before she tried to implement it more widely (Hall and Hord 2011: 226). By piloting the initiative first, she would have the chance to communicate regularly with her team and other schools about the project, and perhaps move more people towards being ready to change, whilst also maintaining the interest of the people who were enthusiastic about, or had agreed to, the project (Reinhardt and Keller 2009). Nevertheless, if more people than she anticipated were keen to participate at the outset, more pilot sites could be proposed, or the project rolled out across all the schools: but it would then be the choice of individuals to come on board rather than pressure being exerted on them to work in this way before they felt ready to do so. Her initiative was not replacing anything, so it was not something that would be phased in as something else was phased out. The option of the 'big bang' approach seemed unattractive, as there was no need for this change to happen quickly, and it was not yet tried and tested, so piloting it first made sense.

Assessing how ready individuals and teams are for change can help you to decide the best way to introduce an innovation.

Having considered these issues, Leila was ready to tell her colleagues about her idea.

Information Giving

People need information about any new way of working, and a part of planning change is to decide what information to give, when, how, and to whom. Kyriakidou (2011) suggests that people often view a proposed change as either attractive or non-engaging, rather than as a threat or an opportunity. This was how Leila felt people would respond to her proposal: it was unlikely to be seen as a threat (although if other team members had been working on ideas this might be seen as a threat to these). The main issue was likely to be whether it would be seen as interesting, or something people particularly wanted to do, and a major part of encouraging people to move towards contemplating or being ready for change would therefore be to make it attractive, or engaging: to sell the idea.

One important part of selling a new idea, as Chapter 3 identified, is to be clear about: exactly what it will involve, why it is happening, why this rather than another approach has been taken, why it is being done now, how it will affect individuals' work, whether people have the skills they will need, and if not whether they will be given support and training to enable them to acquire these skills (Kotter 1995, Giangreco and Peccei 2005, Golden 2006, Pare et al. 2011). If people are at the pre-contemplation or contemplation stage of readiness for change, the information given should be aimed at convincing them to consider or accept the idea of change. If they are already ready for change but awaiting the rolling out of the new way of working, the way information is given and what is said needs to help them to maintain their enthusiasm until the project starts. One of Leila's key points was that this innovation was, at this point in time, going to be piloted by herself and a colleague, but that if anyone else wanted to participate, that would be even better. She aimed to avoid making people feeling coerced to participate before they were ready, but equally to encourage anyone who did want to join in to do so. She also emphasised that the initial plan was a pilot, so that it could be evaluated and tweaked before investing more time and resources in it. She explained exactly what she was planning, how this would work, what organisational requirements it would meet, why she had chosen this approach, and floated the idea that she hoped to make a closer link with a particular school through the project. The information she gave was met with general assent but not great enthusiasm, although afterwards two of her colleagues asked if they could set up a second pilot at another school, mainly because they saw this as a way of maintaining a link they had with that school.

Leila asked if people would be happy to provide occasional cover for those involved in the pilot. Most people nodded (which might or might not, as Chapter 5 will discuss, signal actual agreement), and no one refused. The response confirmed what Leila had suspected: that people would be relatively indifferent to the idea, but might become more enthusiastic as time went by, depending on how the pilots progressed. She was also interested to see that her idea about creating closer links with a particular school or schools being attractive to some staff had been justified, and brought two people to the stage of being prepared to participate in the initiative.

In addition to what information is given, who delivers it is also important. Chapter 3 discussed the importance of identifying key players in change, and if people have been selected as key players because they are seen as credible, liked, and trusted it may be useful to involve them in information giving (Golden 2006). Leila hoped that she was seen as trustworthy person, and a credible source of information, but she also had as her ally a nurse who had worked in the team for many years and was generally very well respected. She felt that having her backing, and assistance in presenting the initial ideas about the initiative, was an advantage.

Information giving is likely to be more successful if the message is customised to the audience (Golden 2006, Paton and McCalman 2008: 50).

It may be difficult to do this when you almost inevitably have a mixed audience, but gauging the dominant view, or mood, should influence how you present information, and the main points you emphasise. With her colleagues, Leila emphasised that this project would in part fulfil some of the team's required work, and was an idea that they could use and develop, rather than having activities that would meet organisational goals imposed on them. Although she was enthusiastic about her project, she sensed that for some of the team this was just one more idea that would go nowhere, or would tick a box for a while before something else came along (Welch and McCarville 2003, Parkin 2009: 7). She felt that if she seemed naively over enthusiastic it might fuel this perception, and therefore tried to present a balanced, well-thought, and logical plan. When she spoke to staff at the schools, although she gave the same basic message, she placed more emphasis on engaging with parents than meeting her own organisation's requirements. She was also aware that the information devised to invite parents to attend would require a further approach that was fairly informal and non-threatening (an opportunity for discussion and sharing ideas, not criticizing what they did). In her planning, she identified that parents were the real key players, because unless they chose to attend the drop-in sessions, the initiative would fail. The information sent to them was therefore perhaps even more vital than the information given to her colleagues and school staff.

The amount and timing of the information that people receive, as well as the information itself, can influence whether or not they support a change in practice. A balance has to be achieved between information overload and not giving adequate or frequent enough information to sustain interest. After she had given the initial information about her project to the school nurses' team, Leila suggested that she provide updates at the team's monthly meetings and in the monthly newsletters, which seemed manageable, but not too intrusive. There was an option to provide email updates, but as most people attended the meetings, or saw the newsletter, she thought that this would only increase their mail load and not be read. For the school, she planned to provide updates at staff meetings, and for parent newsletters. To remind parents of the drop-in sessions, she intended to have posters on display at all the school entrances on the days the sessions ran. The schools she hoped to involve used a text messaging system for events and she planned to ask if the drop-in sessions could be announced by text on the day before they were held and on the morning itself, to serve as a timely reminder for parents.

The information that is given about an innovation should target everyone who will need to be on board for change to happen.

Setting Timescales

Planning the timescale for change is useful, so that you do not delay for ever, but at the same time give yourself enough time to get everything done that needs doing before the new way of working commences, and at each stage of it (Schifalacqua et al. 2009). It is also expedient to decide when any pilot stage will end and formal evaluations take place, so that you think realistically about how long it will take for the project to be adequately established to have made a difference, and for meaningful judgments to be able to be made about it. Leila estimated that she could hold the first drop-in meeting about a month after getting permission for the project, and doing this at the start of a new school term seemed a sensible time. Running the pilot project for a term before evaluating it would be appropriate: longer would be too long, because if changes were needed they should be made sooner rather than later, and enthusiasm for expanding the project might be lost if the results from the first phase were not evident. If the pilot lasted less time, there would not really be an opportunity to iron out any problems that occurred and establish the program. She also felt that a term would allow a number of staff to dip into the project and get an idea of what was happening, and it formed a natural timeframe in the life of the school and school nursing services.

As well as having a start date and a date by which you aim to achieve your goal, it can be helpful to have timetabled stages along the way to enable you to see what you have achieved, and whether you are on track, even if you have not completed the task yet (Schifalacqua et al. 2009). Sometimes you cannot set the final target date until you have achieved some intermediate milestones, so having dates for earlier stage goals can be useful (Clarke 2001). If the change process you are initiating is likely to be long, having a staged timetable can help you to see whether things are on track, and maintain motivation, even when the end still seems some way off. Although Leila's project was relatively straightforward, and she expected it to be rolled out fairly quickly, she devised a timetable that included the preparatory work until the first drop-in session for parents, when the pilot would complete, and when a decision would be made about next steps.

It is important that your timetable is realistic. Sometimes things can sound as if they will be easier than they actually are, and thinking through exactly what you will have to do to achieve each part of your plan can help you to make it achievable. At the same time, although having a timetable should help you to keep your project on track, unavoidable delays may happen, and unplanned events creep in (Hall and Hord 2011: 145). Any timetable needs to be flexible: if one goal gets delayed then the other dates will probably need to be altered in light of this, instead of striving for the unachievable. If you find that you have underestimated the time you need for any stage, it is better to re-plan than to try to do an impossible catch-up task, become disheartened, and give up.

Action planning is a way of documenting the plans and processes that will be needed to make something, in this case change, happen. There is no one correct way to present an action plan, but documenting it in tabular format can make clear at a glance what you are meant to be doing, show where you are at, what still needs to be done, and what you have achieved. How you make an action plan, or plan for change, is a personal choice, but an example from Leila's work is seen in Figure 4.2. The statements of what you will do in an action plan may seem quite obvious, but planning the process of change in detail can help you to avoid unexpected pitfalls. Thinking through logically 'what would I need to do in order for that to happen?' and noting everything that will be necessary can mean that you do not suddenly discover that what you had hoped to do cannot be achieved because some crucial resource is missing. It is often useful to divide your project into stages or objectives in order to help you to consider, for each stage: what you aim to achieve, what you will need, who will need to be involved, who will support you, whom you need to convince of the value of changing practice, what is needed for this to happen, how long you expect it will take, and how you will decide if you have achieved it.

Having a plan that details every step of a proposed change, and timescales for these, enables you to see whether you have thought of everything, have the resources and support you will need, and if things are on schedule at any given time.

Planning to Maintain Motivation

The people whom you work with will probably be at different stages of readiness for change. How you will sustain the motivation of those who are ready to move forward when there are not yet enough of them, or whilst the practicalities of the initiative are still being explored or set up, merits consideration. Leila was aware that her colleagues who were going to be involved in the pilots were now all keen to start the initiative, but that final approval from her manager and the schools concerned was still needed. Leila made sure that her plan of the run-up to rolling out the new way of working showed when the meetings with the manager and schools concerned would happen, when letters would be written, posters would be designed, and when she hoped the drop-in sessions would begin. By sharing this with her colleagues, and keeping them involved in the preparatory activities, she aimed to sustain their interest.

Aim: To make information on healthy eating available to the parents of primary school children

Objective	How this will be achieved and by whom	Resources needed	How achievement of the objective will be evaluated	Target date
To hold weekly drop-in sessions for parents	Discuss possibilities with Head Teachers of chosen schools (Leila and Debra for St James', Gina and Steve for Ashdown)	Time	Meeting held: yes/no	23rd November
	Book room at school (Leila, Steve)	Time and room	Room available: yes/no	30th November
	Send letter to parents	Time, writing resources, school liaison to send letters out	Letter sent: yes/no	3rd January
	Run sessions (Leila and Debra for St James', Gina and Steve for Ashdown)	Room at school, information leaflets, staff (one nurse per session per school), posters and text reminders	Note if any sessions did not run on either site, and why	29th March
To provide an, opportunity for parents to discuss nutritional issues	Sessions to run with no specific agenda, but with written information and a school nurse available. Facilitate discussion in a way that is not critical or threatening, and encourages discussion with staff and other parents (Leila, Debra, Gina, Steve, and others who are available to assist)	Room at school, leaflets, staff who are willing to work in this way; Opportunity for other staff to join groups to gain experience or confidence; Evaluation questionnaires to ascertain parent and staff views	Evaluation questionnaires to staff and parents; Discussion with team members who have participated; Informal discussions/observations with parents during the process	29th March
To give parents a chance to suggest ways in which information sharing and support regarding healthy eating could be improved	Invite parents to share their views during sessions, and on evaluation questionnaires (Leila, Debra, Gina, Steve)	Parents being at sessions; Evaluation questionnaires	Evaluation questionnaire; Comments from parents during sessions	29th March

Figure 4.2 Action plan

As well as planning ways to maintain motivation whilst everything is being put in place for a new initiative to begin, it is worth considering how you will maintain the motivation of those who are on board, whilst also recruiting more support once the change is rolled out. Leila's plans included how she would keep those who were participating in her initial pilots on board, and prevent their enthusiasm being eroded by anyone who opposed her idea. Her intention was to include feedback from both the pilot sites at the team meetings and in the newsletter updates, so that they all felt continued ownership of the project, and that their contributions were valued. She also planned to meet regularly with the team at the second school in the early stages of the project, to get updates on how things were going, and to provide any support or input that they needed. Recruiting more support would be achieved through opportunities for others to work on the project, and providing feedback to the team as a whole during the pilots. These opportunities might also give Leila informal feedback on people's level of enthusiasm or desire to participate, so that she could gauge their ongoing readiness for change.

Prochaska and Diclemante's (1992) fifth or final stage of change is that of maintaining change. This is discussed in more detail in Chapter 10, but unless change is sustained (provided that there is not a good reason why it should be abandoned), then the effort devoted to implementing it is time that you could have used on something else. Despite being the last, this can be the most challenging stage of change, and should feature in your plans. At this stage, it was too early for Leila to think of this in much detail, because she was not yet convinced her idea would work. Her plans were tentative, but she was aware that, in the fullness of time, if things did work out, she would have to consider ways of maintaining the new way of working, so that it did not become something that, as some of the team seemed to expect, was good whilst it lasted, but not a long-term achievement.

Summary

The quality of the planning that precedes change often affects how smoothly the change is implemented, and how successful it is. Planning includes thinking about the human and material factors that may drive or restrain change, readiness of people and organisations for change, and the best way of introducing change. Planning when, how, and by whom information will be given, the timetable for change, and how motivation for change will be maintained and developed whilst it is rolled out should also be considered. In most initiatives, it is useful to find a way of documenting your plans, so that you can check that nothing has been missed, can see at a glance whether or not you are on track, and can plan what needs to be done next, and by whom.

During the planning stage, and whilst change is being rolled out, a major consideration is what the barriers to change are likely to be, and how they can be reduced.

Key Points

Successful change requires the forces driving change to be greater than those restraining it.

Driving and restraining forces include human factors, resources, and training needs.

Assessing how ready people are for change gives an indication of whether an innovation should go ahead.

How people are told about change affects their acceptance of it: messages need to be customised to each audience.

Having a clear plan for implementing change makes it easier to ensure that nothing is missed.

CASE STUDY

Sami is a link nurse for infection control in a general medical ward. The hospital infection control team have recently developed a new protocol for the administration of intravenous drugs that is about to be piloted on four wards in the surgical directorate. If the pilot has the expected outcome, the protocol will be rolled out across the NHS Trust and Sami will be responsible for implementing it on his ward. In the run-up to what he anticipates will be a requirement for him to introduce the new way of working, he has been thinking about the best way to approach this.

What Driving and Restraining Forces Were There Likely to Be?

Whilst the protocol was being developed, Sami began to think about what the driving and restraining forces for changing practice on his ward might be.

If there was a requirement for people to adopt the new protocol, this could serve as both a driving and restraining force. It could be a driving force because failure to comply would mean that the required way of working was being breached, and disciplinary action could, in theory at least, be taken. This links with a power coercive approach to change and might mean that people complied out of fear, rather than understanding why they should do things differently. It might also create resentment, and mean that the new way of working was used when people felt they were being watched, but not otherwise. Sami wanted to look at other ways in which he could increase people's motivation to change their practice, as well as reduce the restraining forces.

Sami thought that if people understood why the new protocol was being introduced, and what the advantages might be, for staff and patients, it would reduce the restraining forces and increase the driving forces for change. The stated reason for the new protocol was to reduce infection and increase efficiency. He thought that this would be more likely to be a driving force for his ward if he could find information on whether there had been any specific problems with the administration of intravenous drugs that necessitated the protocol, and how the new approach improved things, in terms of infection control and efficiency. He therefore asked the person leading the initiative for information about the reason for the new protocol, and why the new approach was thought to be superior to what was currently done. He also felt that the efficiency argument would be more convincing if his colleagues could see the new way of working in action.

What Resources Would Be Needed?

The resources needed for the new way of working to be introduced would be time for training the staff. No new equipment or supplies would be needed, but Sami thought it would be useful to have some printed reminders and copies of the protocol to laminate and put up in the treatment room, where the staff prepared the drugs. Otherwise, people forgetting about the new way of working on a busy shift could easily become a restraining force.

What Education or Training Would Be Needed?

The staff would have to learn a new protocol for administering intravenous drugs, which would require not only some training, but for them to remember to do things in the new way. This could be a restraining force, because of the time and effort required. Sami considered whether he could reduce this by enabling the staff to gain an informal preview of what might be required by them visiting the surgical wards where the pilots were happening. This had the potential to reduce the apparent threat of a new way of working, as people would be able to see what was really required. If the procedure was said to be more efficient, seeing it rather than just being told about it was likely to be more convincing.

What Stage of Readiness for Change Were People Likely to Be at?

Sami thought that there was likely to be relatively low readiness for change amongst his colleagues, as infection linked to intravenous drug administration was rarely seen in his ward. There were likely to be a few people who easily became ready for change when they heard about the new way of working, but the vast majority would be at the pre-contemplation stage, when they saw no need for change, or at the contemplation stage, when they would be prepared to listen and consider it, but would not yet be really convinced that this was necessary. He would need to introduce the new protocol in a way that helped people to move from pre-contemplation or contemplation to readiness for change.

What Would Be the Best Way of Introducing the New Way of Working?

The Trust as a whole was piloting the new way of working and if this showed a good outcome, all wards and departments would be required to implement it, but Sami thought that enabling his staff to visit the pilot wards and see the scheme in action would help them to see the pilot as real. He also planned to make sure that he had the findings from the pilot to share with his colleagues, so that they knew that it really had been piloted and evaluated.

When, How, and to Whom Would Sami Give Information?

Sami decided that he would begin giving information to staff on his ward as soon as the pilot was established (about six weeks into it) so that people had time to consider the new way of working, ask questions, and so that he had time to work on helping people to move to readiness for change. If he did this earlier, and the new way of working did not ultimately happen, he felt that it would create unnecessary confusion.

Sami wanted to introduce the idea of the new protocol at a ward meeting, but as not everyone could attend, he would also put the information in the communication book and on the staff email. He would follow this up by a list of the staff being placed in the office so that they could sign up for visits to the pilot sites to see the new way of working in action.

Although Sami would, of necessity, be leading this change in practice, he wanted information to come from others as well, preferably those with experience in the new way of working. He not only wanted his colleagues to visit the pilot sites to see the new way of working, but also to enable them to ask questions and discuss it with people who were actually using it. In addition, he thought it would be useful to ask those who had been to the pilot wards to feed back at a staff meeting in the six weeks before the new protocol was rolled out on his ward.

What Would the Timetable for Change Be?

Once the new protocol was introduced, there would be very little option for Sami timetabling an approach to change, as everyone would be expected to work in the new way almost at once. He therefore timetabled information giving activities, and preparations for the new way of working, whilst the pilot was running. He scheduled the point six weeks into the pilot to determine whether it was likely to be adopted, and then planned to use the final six weeks until the end of the pilot to let the staff in his ward know about it – why it was happening, what the consequence might be for them – and set up opportunities for all staff members to visit the pilot wards. When the pilot was complete, and the new protocol ready to be rolled out, he planned to have two weeks for final staff training, creating reminders, laminating them, and putting them up. At this stage, he could not put precise dates to all these events, as he was not certain of how things would progress, but he wanted to be sure that he had listed all the requisite tasks and approximately when, and in what sequence, they would happen.

How Would Sami Maintain Motivation for Change?

Although Sami was still at the planning stage of a change in practice that might never get beyond the pilot stage, he began to consider how the new protocol could become embedded in practice. As there was no particular equipment needed, supplies would not be an issue. The ward was generally too busy for anyone to closely monitor what was happening, so checking on whether people actually worked in this way was not viable. His idea was that he would evaluate the success of the implementation of the protocol by discussing with staff whether they found it achievable and what the pros and cons of it were. He would informally check on what people did, but this would not give him a complete picture of what was happening. The main way in which he felt he could obtain an accurate picture of whether or not the protocol was being used, and to what effect, was to keep communication channels open, and encourage honest feedback. This would also mean that the new protocol remained in focus after it was introduced, and he was seen to be taking an interest and acting on any difficulties encountered. It would also mean that if genuine difficulties did exist with the new way of working, he could feed these back to the infection control team.

GUIDED WORK

This section revisits the learning outcomes covered in the chapter. You may want to complete it alone, or with colleagues.

1. Identify driving and restraining forces that might affect the success of an innovation.

Identify a change in practice that you would be interested in making in your workplace. List

*   The practical driving forces;
*   The people-centred driving forces;
*   The practical restraining forces;
*   The people-centred restraining forces.

Consider whether the driving forces would outweigh or be outweighed by the restraining forces. Is there anything you could do to reduce the restraining forces and build on the driving forces?

2. Understand how individual and team readiness for change influence its success.

Using the innovation that you identified above

*   Think about which members of your team would be likely to be at the pre-contemplation, contemplation, or determination for change stage.
*   Consider how these people might influence others, and the effect that this would have on the readiness for change of the team as a whole.
*   Decide whether the best way of introducing the new way of working would be by a pilot, phasing it in, or using a 'big bang' approach.

3. Appreciate how different approaches to giving information about change may be successful with different audiences.

Decide who would need to be informed of the change in practice you identified above. For each individual or group, state

- When you would give them information.
- What information you would provide them with.
- How you would provide it.

4. Develop a plan for change that includes human and practical elements.

For the change in practice that you have identified above, design an action plan that includes

- The practical steps that will need to be taken.
- Who will need to be consulted with or involved at each stage.
- How people's opinions, questions, or concerns about the innovation will be identified.

5. Set a realistic timescale for introducing innovation.

On your action plan, add a timescale for when you would expect to begin and complete each stage.

Additional Resources

Action planning:
http://www.institute.nhs.uk/quality_and_service_improvement_tools/quality_and_service_improvement_tools/action_planning.html

Force field analysis:
http://www.practical-management-skills.com/change-management-tools.html

Readiness for change:
http://www.klr.com/articles/Articles_ChangeManagement_change_readiness_assessment.pdf

5

Barriers to Change

Chapter Learning Outcomes

After studying this chapter, the reader will be able to:

- Understand the potential value of resistance to change
- Recognise a range of possible causes of resistance to change
- Consider how individual and group resistance to change can influence one another
- Appreciate the significance of opinion leaders and key stakeholders in overcoming resistance to change
- Plan innovation in a manner that is likely to minimise resistance to it.

Summary

This chapter focuses on the causes of resistance to change, and how it can be reduced or managed. It begins with a discussion of the value of some degree of resistance to change and the importance of trying to ascertain the real reasons why people may oppose change. This is followed by an exploration of how individual and corporate experience history of change, other concurrent or recent changes, the basis of the evidence for a need for change, losses associated with change, individual circumstances and lifestyles, established routines or practice, and apprehension about a new way of working that can affect the implementation of change. It highlights how opposition by key individuals and groups can influence the success of change, and the role of patients as key stakeholders and opinion leaders in whether or not change succeeds.

Rob works in a residential unit for 20 adults with severe learning disabilities. At a recent service review, it was recommended that the staff should improve their knowledge of alternative methods of communicating with the residents. Rob thought that the best way to address this recommendation was for small groups of staff to each learn one new approach to communication. This would mean that a core group of staff were able to use each method, and could support and teach others in working with residents who used, or might usefully use, that approach. His idea was that each group would also make an information file so that a practical and user-friendly resource about a range of methods of communication was available in the unit.

After discussing this with a couple of members of staff, who seemed to think it was a good idea, Rob put his plan forward at a team meeting. There was not a great deal of response to his suggestion. One person stated that she had tried to learn other ways of communicating before and had found it very difficult. Another two commented that making the files would be time consuming and that no one would have time to look in them once they were complete. Someone else said that they did not really think that any action was needed, as the next review would not be for two years, and things could have changed by then. The people Rob had already discussed the project with did not say anything. Rob listened to what was said, and then invited the staff to come up with other ideas to meet the requirements of the review. As no one had any immediate suggestions, Rob asked them to think about it for a week, after which they would have another meeting to share their thoughts.

Rob was disappointed with how things had gone. The unit had to show that they were addressing this issue, and he had thought that sharing out the work of learning about alternative approaches to communication would make it manageable. He was a little disheartened that his idea had not been well received, especially as the two people who had seemed to approve of it when he spoke to them had not supported him.

Although people opposing or resisting an innovation that you suggest can be disappointing, almost all change encounters some opposition. Chapter 4 discussed force field analysis (weighing up the forces that may drive or restrain change) (Lewin 1951, Parkin 2009: 152–153), and the need to consider individual and group readiness when planning change (Holt et al. 2007, Pare et al. 2011). A part of this is thinking about the things, which may mean that people resist a new way of working (restraining forces, and factors reducing readiness for change), as they are likely to prevent an otherwise well-planned initiative from happening. Rob therefore now needed to think about why people had not embraced his idea, and whether there was any way of reducing his team's resistance to the change he had suggested by lessening the restraining forces as well as by increasing the driving forces and their readiness for change.

Resistance as a Positive

Resistance to change if often portrayed as a negative entity, with connotations of people being stuck in their ways, difficult, and preventing practice from moving forward. If you have had an idea that could improve practice, or have devised a solution to an identified problem, people being negative about your thoughts can feel exactly like this. It was, broadly speaking, how Rob felt: the unit was required to do something, he had thought of an idea to meet the requirement, a couple of people had agreed with him, and now they were saying nothing and everyone else was making difficulties.

However, although it is unlikely to feel this way if it is your project that is being opposed, resistance to change is a very understandable and, in principle, sensible thing. Change alters the status quo; it creates uncertainty about what people are expected to do and can expect others to do, and reduces their control over situations (Welch and McCarville 2003). Instead of wondering why change is resisted, it may be more realistic to ask why people would want to accept it (Price 2008). This can be difficult to do, especially if your idea has fallen on unenthusiastic ears, but it can help you to clarify what the positive aspects of the change you are suggesting are, and why people might want to participate.

People questioning or opposing your plans can also be useful because it makes you think things through thoroughly. If no one questions your idea, it may mean that possible pitfalls or problems are missed (McDonnell et al. 2006). Although it may not feel that way when it is your idea at stake, other people challenging you can safeguard against over optimism and make you consider every aspect of a situation, so that the new way of working is more robust in the long term (de Jager 2001, Fronda and Moriceau 2008, Wright 2010). People questioning your ideas can also stop something from happening that, although it looks and sounds good at first, is never going to work or might even be dangerous. A culture in which every idea was immediately adopted without question would be as problematic as one in which people resist all change. A healthy organisation needs a certain amount of scepticism and questioning so that it knows why it does the things it does, and thinks things through before implementing them (Parkin 2009: 159).

It is, nonetheless, OK to go away and sulk over a coffee and cake for a while before you come round to this way of thinking.

Resistance to change can be discouraging, but it also serves a useful protective function.

Recognising Resistance

When you introduce the idea of change, resistance to it may be as easy to spot, but it may not, and it is useful to think about what individuals seem to be saying, what groups appear to be saying, how the two are linked, and what may be being left unsaid.

Individuals can be strongly influenced by the groups they belong to, and, as Chapter 3 identified, opinion leaders can easily sway the opinion of others (Grol and Grimashaw 2003, Scott et al. 2003). How individuals' resistance may influence group resistance, and the vice versa, is therefore an important consideration in managing change (Qian and Daniels 2008, Cameron and Green 2009: 9, Erwin and Garman 2010). Rob realised that he had been a little naïve in his expectation that the two people who had apparently supported his idea when he spoke to them would actually do so, and do so in public. Whilst they might think his idea was workable, when others had opposed it, it was not completely surprising that they had not spoken out. They might also have been persuaded by others to rethink their initial acceptance, either because of the arguments people presented, or because of who they were. It could equally be that they had only ever agreed with him because that was the easiest option at the time, and they were in fact fairly ambivalent about the idea, and would go with whatever was decided. As the person whose idea this had been, and the one likely to be required to make changes, Rob had interpreted their responses as support, when in fact they might merely have signalled a lack of opposition or neutrality.

When Someone Seems to Support Your Idea for Innovation, Ask Yourself:

What or who might influence them to change their mind?
Do they agree, or are they being polite?
Do they agree, or can they not be bothered to argue?
Do they agree, or do they just not disagree?

Apathy can be the most difficult type of resistance to deal with (Giangreco and Peccei 2005). People who are apathetic about change do not really oppose it, it is simply not something that they think matters particularly, or that they are interested enough in to make time in their days to do. For the same reason, they may not feel inclined to argue about it, or express their views, because it is not important enough. Convincing them to join in a change initiative may be much harder than overcoming strongly felt, stated, objections to a new way of working. Although change can feel threatening for individuals and organisations, Kyriakidou (2011) suggests that people are more likely to view a proposed change as non-engaging than as a threat. Where people are apathetic, they do not oppose change so much as see it as non-engaging, and making an initiative seem more interesting or important can be more difficult than overcoming specific objections to it.

Resistance to change may be active or passive (Parkin 2009:155). People who openly challenge your ideas may be off-putting, but you know what has been said, by whom, and what their objections are, which means that you can think about how to handle them. Opposition that is not openly stated can be much harder to address. Whilst some people who do not state their opposition to an idea will not claim to support it either, others may appear to support an innovation, promise to participate, and then fail to do so. Rob realised that apathy and silent opposition were probably going to be important considerations in his attempt to introduce a new way of working, and that he would have to try to gauge how and why it existed, and how he could best address it. One of the unit staff spoke Makaton and British Sign Language, and Rob had supposed that she, knowing the importance of these other forms of communication, would support his idea. However, although she had said nothing, she had looked stony and unenthusiastic during the meeting, and he now felt that her unspoken disapproval or failure to engage would affect his plans. In addition to her own opposition, she was likely to be an opinion leader within the team, because of her history in the organisation and her status as the expert in communication. Her unspoken opposition would therefore need to be handled appropriately. He also realised that, even if she did openly oppose his plans, she might not state what her real opposition was about.

An apparent lack of opposition to change does not necessarily mean that none exists.

Knowing What People Are Really Opposed to

People resist change for a number of reasons, and whilst what a person says they object to is often exactly what they do object to, this may not always be the case. Finding the real reason why people are opposing a proposed change is a vital part of addressing resistance, because otherwise you may deal with what they say is the problem, but be no closer to gaining their support.

Rob had assumed that the person who spoke Makaton and British Sign Language would know the importance of these forms of communication, and support his suggestion. However, on reflection, he realised that at present she had an important role as the expert in alternative forms of communication, and, if the work was divided up and expertise shared as he proposed, her informal, but universally acknowledged, role would be lost (Carroll and Quijada 2004: ii17). However, it was unlikely that she would say: 'I don't want that to happen because I am the expert in alternative methods of communication, everyone knows that, and I won't be any more if this goes ahead.' It was much more likely that she would appear to resist change for other reasons, or fail to engage with it. Unless he thought about and addressed the real, but probably unspoken, problem, he might spend time tweaking various parts of his idea, to no avail.

It may be something not directly related to the new way of working that concerns people the most. Rob realised that the two people who had cited the extra information gathering and learning they would have to do as problematic might in fact be concerned about competing commitments, rather than the activity itself (Kegan and Lahey 2001). Both were completing National Vocational Qualifications (NVQ), and were possibly concerned about managing the work from his proposal in addition to their existing studies, rather than really thinking the idea was not, in principle, a good one. He thought that perhaps he should have suggested that they explore whether they would be able to use the work they did for the initiative he was suggesting for their NVQ studies. He had also suggested, to try to make the initiative more interesting, that staff could visit a communication centre to learn about alternative options for communicating, and perhaps attend study days or workshops about the approaches they each chose. The person who had said that this seemed a lot of work for something two years away, which might not even be required worked very limited hours, and Rob wondered if the likelihood of things changing over the next two years might not really have been her main objection. She might have been more concerned that she would be obliged to attend events that created problems with her working hours and personal arrangements.

As well as finding out what aspect of change, or what collateral effects of change, are a concern for individuals, it is useful to try to identify whether it is the idea behind the new way of working, or how it is being introduced, that people oppose (Parkin 2009: 159–160). Rob wondered whether, because the change was being instigated because of an external review and recommendation, staff might see what they were being asked to do as a criticism of their practice. His approach had, he thought, perhaps come across as a punitive managerial imposition. He recognised that he had not really commended his staff for the fact that they generally communicated well with the residents, and that one of them spoke Makaton and British Sign Language. He hoped, at the next meeting, to focus on developing practice, rather than correcting shortfalls, and involve his team more in thinking of ideas, taking an active part in, and owning any new way of working (Jimmieson et al. 2008, Paton and McCalman 2008: 29, Ludwick and Doucette 2009). There was no real history of the unit staff thinking about, and designing, new ways of working, so Rob had not really considered this. However, he now thought that he could perhaps use this opportunity to introduce his team to developing the skills and confidence to reflect on their practice, values, and priorities, and from this look to design and trial new approaches to practice, rather than imposing his views on them. This has links with the concepts of emancipatory and transformational practice development described in Chapter 1 (Manley and McCormack 2003, Wilson and McCormack 2006, Dewing 2010, Walsh et al. 2011), which was the direction in which Rob would ideally like his workplace to move.

Having begun to consider the reasons why his team had not appeared as enthusiastic about his idea as he had hoped, Rob looked in more detail at what specific issues might be barriers to his team accepting the idea of developing the way they communicated with residents.

Addressing resistance to change can mean looking beyond what people say is the cause of their opposition, and finding the real cause.

What Do People Oppose in Change?

What is changing, or how their role or status will change
What is changing, or how this will affect other aspects of their work or life
What is changing, or how change is being introduced

History

The culture and history of a workplace are likely to influence how the staff in it respond to suggestions for change (Parkin 2009: 105, Hall and Hord 2011: 21). Although there is not complete consensus on what 'organisational culture' means (Scott et al. 2003), it is generally thought to include the social environment, attitudes to work, expected behaviours, beliefs, relationships, and the history of change in the organisation (Cameron and Green 2009: 255–256, Parkin 2009: 105). Thinking about your workplace culture in relation to change includes considering whether it is somewhere where developing practice is the accepted norm, and, if so, how this is usually approached.

Some workplaces regularly engage in change, however, the culture that this creates may exist anywhere on a continuum from practitioner-led emancipatory or transformational practice development to purely technical developments (Manley and McCormack 2003, Wilson and McCormack 2006, Dewing 2010, Walsh et al. 2011). In other situations, a history of constant but apparently random, pointless, or unsuccessful changes can mean that teams do not take suggestions for innovation seriously (Welch and McCarville 2003). There are also organisations or teams that rarely encounter innovations or changes in practice.

The culture of change in an organisation or team includes the way in which the group as a whole have experienced change in the past, but also individuals' experiences of change. These may be general experiences of change, or relate to the particular change being suggested (Golden 2006, McCabe 2010). As well as considering a team or organisation's past history of change, it is useful to think about their recent history. If this includes a successful change in practice, you may be able to bolster your initiative by taking advantage of the impetus that it has created, especially if it is related to your project (Scott et al. 2003). Alternatively, if a change in practice has recently been unsuccessful, you may want to wait until everyone forgets their negative feelings about that before you present another new idea (Scott et al. 2003, Golden 2006).

Rob thought about the culture of his workplace, and, although the team provided good care, and made small innovations from time to time, these were usually projects with individual residents, rather than larger, whole team, efforts. So, the way he was suggesting that his idea should be implemented was quite different from their usual approach to change. Oakland and Tanner (2007) and Cameron and Green (2009: 260) suggest that change is more likely to be embraced if it builds on the positive aspects of the current workplace culture. Rob wondered if he should have acknowledged that the unit staff often did new things with individual residents, and suggested that they could develop their skills in communication on this type of individual basis, with particular residents' communication needs as the focus. This might have made it seem closer to their usual way of working. He also realised that whilst the staff gave good care, the culture of the unit was very much that work was for work time, and a means of employment, not something that should encroach on the rest of their lives. He thought that perhaps he could have made it clearer that they would not be expected to do the work on new communication methods in their own time, and explained how he planned to free up work time for them to achieve this.

Rob also recalled that following a previous review, four years earlier (before he was in post), the team had been asked to change the way they documented the administration of medication. During the changeover to the new documentation, there had been several medication errors, which had been informally blamed on the new system. Thus, there might be some residual fear or opposition to changes arising from reviews, because the previous one was perceived to have created difficulties. One person who had not said anything, but had looked rather dismissive throughout the discussion, had probably been involved in those incidents. Rob thought that perhaps he should have acknowledged the unit's past experience of change arising from reviews, explained why this one was unlikely to carry the same risks, and outlined the benefits that it was expected bring.

Thinking about how individuals and groups have experienced change in the past is useful in planning innovation.

Evidence of Potential Benefit

The apparent benefits of change understandably influence people's acceptance of it. Chapter 2 discussed how presenting the reasons and evidence for a proposed change can increase people's acceptance of it. However, it is not just whether you have evidence that change is necessary that affects its acceptance or otherwise. It depends on whether those concerned find that evidence convincing, important, or feel that the outcome is likely to be beneficial. The unit staff acknowledged that few of them could use alternative forms of communication, but there was a feeling that the person who could do so helped the others to communicate with residents where necessary, and that this approach worked well. As a result, they did not really feel convinced that everyone needed to develop such skills, or that doing so would particularly enhance the care they gave. Rob felt that he had not really provided them with any evidence to challenge that view, or to suggest that their efforts to gain new skills would enhance day-to-day practice. Although he had given a reason for the proposed change, this had included little of the empirical rational approach (Chin and Benne 1985) (discussed in Chapter 3). The reason he had given had been based on an external demand, not evidence of how residents or staff would benefit from the new way of working.

Rob now thought about how he could best explain the benefits that he felt more staff being able to use alternative communication methods would have. He decided to search for research and other evidence on the subject so as to confirm whether or not his suggestion actually was sensible. If it was, this would enable him to provide a summary of the existing evidence to his team. In addition, to make this more relevant to day to day practice on the unit, he also considered putting together a list of situations that sometimes occurred with existing residents, and asking staff to reflect on these, and use this as a platform to explore how different ways of communicating might have be useful. As well as making these suggestions relevant to the unit, it would provide him with a means of encouraging staff to begin the process of reflecting on their current work, why they worked in this way, and developing ideas for innovations. This would be a start point for moving towards a more transformational than technical approach to developing practice (Dewing 2010, Walsh et al. 2011).

Rob thought that his approach to information giving so far had tended towards the power coercive approach to change (Chin and Benne 1985), with reward or punishment for working in a new way being the focus (Cameron and Green 2009: 19–25). However, it seemed that this approach was not particularly effective, especially as the threat of not changing their practice was seen by staff as relatively weak. One person had stated that if they did nothing the unit could not be closed down, suggesting that although the change was apparently required, the threat of anything happening if they did not act on the recommendations from the review was fairly empty. Rob began to think about how, even if he did have to use some element of coercion, he could make this more attractive, or positive, perhaps in terms of developing additional skills enabling people to gain certification in using alternative methods of communication, take on a teaching role outside the organisation, or being considered for a higher grade. His intention now was to enable people to feel that they were being offered the potential for material or status-based rewards for their efforts, rather than being threatened with punishment or censure if they did not comply (Chin and Benne 1985, Cameron and Green 2009: 19–24).

Information Giving: Things to Consider

What reason are you giving for suggesting change?
What benefits are you highlighting for patients/clients?
What benefits are you highlighting for staff?
What benefits are you highlighting for the organisation?
What evidence can you provide to demonstrate these benefits?
Is this message likely to appeal to your audience?

Even when there is evidence that change will bring some benefits or rewards, for it to be attractive the benefits have to outweigh the threats, so identifying the benefits alone may not be enough (Erwin and Garman 2010). To try to reduce or address resistance to change, it is almost always useful to include elements of the normative re-educative approach to change (Chin and Benne 1985) (discussed in Chapter 3). In this approach, the social and cultural implications of change are the central considerations, and the focus is on the meaning of change for individuals and groups. A part of this is considering what people may lose because of a change in practice.

Giving information on the benefits of change will be of limited value in overcoming resistance if these do not outweigh the threats that change creates.

Change and Loss

When things change, it can mean that people lose something, and experiences of change can therefore be accompanied by feelings of loss (Austin and Currie 2003, Scott et al. 2003, Price 2008, Hall and Hord 2011: 84). Change often requires people to stop doing what they do well, enjoy doing, or feel confident in doing, and to do something else instead (Hall and Hord 2011: 84). It can also affect the role or status of an individual or group (Parkin 2009: 159). This may be a formal role, or something informal but nonetheless important, such as how a person is viewed, and the perceptions that they and others have of their knowledge, expertise, skills, or connections (Carroll and Quijada 2004: ii17). The person in Rob's team who spoke Makaton and British Sign Language had an important, but unofficial, role as the expert in alternative methods of communication, which she enjoyed and which gave her a sense of worth and reward in her work. This role might be threatened by the new way of working. Rob thought that he probably should have spoken to her first, asked her to work with him on developing practice related to communication on the unit, and suggested she take a lead role in facilitating any innovation. This might have lessened her sense of loss and enabled her, in her existing capacity as expert in alternative methods of communication, to be a central part of any new way of working.

Changing the way people work may mean that systems, relationships, demarcations of responsibility, and structures are changed, which can create feelings of insecurity, loss of familiarity, and loss of control (Giangreco and Peccei 2005). Even if a proposed change is not opposed in principle, the feelings of uncertainty that it brings can make embracing it difficult. The change that Rob was proposing did not present any obvious threats to the systems or structure in use, but it probably presented a threat to the unofficial system (that there was no requirement for staff to use alternative approaches to communication). He wondered if people felt that the standard expectation of their working practice was being altered, and whether this created insecurity because the boundaries of acceptable knowledge and skills would change, and the new boundaries be uncertain.

What Loss Might Change Bring?

Loss of established roles
Loss of individual or group status
Loss of familiar systems
Loss of confidence in how to perform procedures
Loss of personal or workplace history
Loss of security over what is expected
Loss of certainty of the outcomes of actions
Loss of sense of control

Seeing change as a process of loss as well as potential gain can be useful in understanding people's responses to it. Worden (1991) and Kubler-Ross (1997) describe how loss requires people to move through stages or tasks before coming to a place where their loss is absorbed and they can move on. Both also acknowledge that grief is not a linear process, but a series of stages between which individuals may move in any direction. In loss associated with change, when people seem to have accepted or begun to move towards readiness to accept the new way of working, they may move in a direction that takes them forward, or back to a disinclination to participate. They may also vacillate between accepting and rejecting change, for instance if they see an idea as essentially good but are not sure how they will fit into it. Rob wondered if this, in part at least, accounted for why the two people who had seemed at first to agree with his idea had not supported him at the meeting.

Loss has been associated with people having to rewrite their personal and corporate narratives, and to find a place for their history and memories in the new order of things (Krueger 2006). Similarly, people who are involved in change may have to rewrite their own narratives in the new way of working. When people suffer loss, it is useful to ensure that what is being lost is still honoured, and valued. An important part of bringing people on board for change can therefore be to help them to find benefits, a place for themselves, and links with what they value from the past, in the new way of working, in a way that outweighs any loss that they feel (Scott et al. 2003, Price 2008, McLean 2011). Rob realised that the person who perhaps felt the most loss was the person who spoke Makaton and British Sign Language. He thought that he should have highlighted her knowledge and expertise and explored with her how any proposed change could use, and build upon this. As things stood, her ten years of being the expert in alternative communication might be seen as being dismissed and devalued. In addition, because the review had suggested that a new way of working was required, it was quite possible that she felt that those conducting the review, and by implication he, had dismissed her knowledge, skills, and input as worthless or inadequate.

Thinking about what individuals and groups may lose as a result of change can be useful in identifying why they may resist innovation.

Established Practice and Routine

Change often means that people have to do things differently, and that established routines, and how things have been done, is lost, which can create a feeling of lack of control (Grol and Grimashaw 2003, Hall and Hord 2011: 84). Although communication with residents was not a routine, and whilst staff currently had difficulties in communicating with some residents, how this was managed was known, and the accepted outcomes were broadly understood. The new approach might create uncertainty over whether the intention was to try different approaches to communication with all the residents who did not communicate verbally, or only with residents who were already known to use alternative means of communicating. If staff used new ways of communicating, they might feel unsure about whether they had really understood the residents, whether they should have, and what the expectation of them was. Rob thought that he should perhaps have given more attention to the detail of how he envisaged staff using their new skills, how they would be introduced in practice, and with which residents.

People's acceptance of a change in practice is likely to be influenced by their confidence in their ability to work in the new way. If individuals feel that they will be unable to perform activities in which they are currently confident and competent, it is likely to be a barrier to them accepting change (Grol and Grimashaw 2003, Cameron and Green 2009: 56). Having to learn new skills or gain new knowledge is time consuming, especially when it replaces something that is currently done almost automatically. Rob's intention had been to reduce the burden of staff having to learn new approaches to communicating by asking everyone to be part of a group that would learn one each. However, he now saw that having to learn any new approach represented a need to gain new skills and knowledge, and that there was a suggestion that in the long term the unit staff would all have to learn a range of ways of communicating. He might have left people feeling uncertain of how they would find time gain the required skills and knowledge, and unsure of whether they would be successful in learning new ways of communicating. Staff who were not used to using alternative ways of communicating might feel uncomfortable using them, fear making mistakes, or creating problems for residents if they were unable to make themselves understood. Rob felt that he could have said a little more about how staff would be supported in their new skills whilst they gained confidence, and thought more about how the new way of working might best be introduced. He now favoured phasing it in, or piloting it, rather than using a big bang approach (Golden 2006, Paton and McCalman 2008:119–120, Pare et al. 2011). The phasing in process might be achieved by starting with a form of communication such as Makaton, which one of the staff was already adept at using, and which a resident on the unit used. The member of staff who already spoke Makaton could support and teach her peers formally, rather than in an ad hoc way, so that change was introduced with support from a trusted colleague, and in a way that valued and utilised her expertise. Alternatively, Rob thought that he might suggest a similar process but as a pilot of staff learning to communicate using Makaton, and evaluating the process and outcomes of that innovation before moving on to learning other methods of communicating. Both these approaches would probably be less threatening than the sudden introduction of a need for all staff members to learn different ways of communicating (Golden 2006, Paton and McCalman 2008:119–120, Pare et al. 2011). It would also allow Rob and the other staff to see some of the benefits and challenges of the new way of working for themselves, and to refine their plans for further communication skill acquisition in light of this.

The outcomes of new practice are usually unknown, and, unless a major problem has created the need for change, the fear of unknown outcomes or consequences may be a barrier to people wanting to alter the way they work. There may be concerns over liability if problems occur, or worries about complaints being made because of a new way of working (Grol and Grimashaw 2003). To allay concerns about what will happen if things do not turn out well or if a complaint is made, it can be useful to clarify where leadership of the change lies, who is accountable for issues arising from it, and who is endorsing it (Grol and Grimashaw 2003). This may mean that individuals are less concerned about the consequences of any problems falling on their heads. Rob was now aware that the outcome of a previous change in response to a review had, in the view of some staff, led to medication errors. He supposed that staff could be concerned that they might not make themselves clearly understood using alternative ways of communicating, or might not interpret residents' responses correctly, and began to think about ways in which he might allay these fears. This included asking staff what they thought the problems might be, looking with them at 'worst case scenarios' and clarifying that the intention was to phase in or pilot the use of new communication systems, with support available, which would minimise the risks.

Planning successful change means thinking about what people will have to do differently, and how this can be made as easy and non-threatening as possible.

Workload

People not having, or not perceiving themselves to have, the time to do things differently is often cited as a reason why change does not go ahead (Oxman and Flottorp 2001, Grol and Grimashaw 2003). Most staff have significant and competing demands on their time, so if there is no obvious harm in the way things are currently done, persuading individuals to spend the time and make the effort to get used to a new way of working can be problematic. Reducing any additional workload occasioned by a change in practice to as little as possible, without losing what needs to be done for change to succeed, whilst also acknowledging the effort required, is one of the skills that may be needed to move people from opposing to accepting a new idea. Rob's idea had been that by sharing the work of learning a range of ways of communicating staff would each have a relatively small workload. However, he now felt that he might not have acknowledged the work that would be needed sufficiently, or explained how he planned to create time in people's everyday work schedules for this.

The time taken to communicate using alternative means on a day-to-day basis might also have been a concern for Rob's team, because whilst in the long-term communication might be more efficient, in the initial stage at least, it would probably take longer. The day-to-day benefits, particularly in the early stages, probably needed to be made clearer. Sometimes seeing the new way of working in action can show its benefits in a way that theory alone cannot, and seeing a trusted colleague working in the new way can be even more convincing than seeing an outsider (Hall and Hord 2011:226). Rob now thought it would be vital to enlist the help of the staff member who spoke Makaton and British Sign Language, to show how, ultimately, communication was likely to be improved, and time saved. In addition, he planned to discuss scenarios from the unit where this would be the case, and look for video clips of scenarios from other situations that illustrated this point.

Client Expectations

Although barriers to change in healthcare are often considered primarily in relation to the staff who will be required to carry out new ways of working, patient or client views and expectations and the views of the general public can be an important part of whether or not change is accepted, and feed into staff acceptance of or opposition to change (Grol and Grimashaw 2003, Scott et al. 2003, van Bokhoven et al. 2003). Whilst Rob had not thought that the change he was suggesting would draw any opposition from the residents, he now considered whether they would find it difficult or frustrating when staff were learning to use new ways of communicating, and if this would feed into staffs' concerns. He also wondered if any families who were themselves disinclined to learn alternative approaches to communication would oppose this approach or feel threatened by the innovation, because it might be seen as implying that they too had to learn it. He thought that he should include this issue in discussions of using new ways of communicating, so that any concerns that staff had over residents or their families' views could be addressed. He also realised that it would probably be beneficial to clarify that no residents would be obliged to use new ways of communicating, if they or their families opposed it. In addition, by introducing the new way of working by piloting it or phasing it in with one or two residents who, and whose families, were interested and willing to try this approach, such concerns might be reduced to a minimum.

Patients or clients are affected by changes in practice: their views about innovations should not be overlooked.

Who Might Affect the Acceptance of Change?

Your managers
Your peers
Patients/clients and their families
The public
Yourself

It can seem strange to think of yourself as being a cause of resistance to change, because if it is your idea, you presumably support it. However, because how change is managed affects resistance to, or acceptance of, it, the ability to be reflective and reflexive, and to think about whether anything in how you are presenting or managing change might be contributing to resistance is important (Moon 2009, Parkin 2009:160). Hall and Hord (2010: 164) identify that regardless of what we actually do or intend to do, what people will respond to is what they think we are doing or intend to do. Although Rob had intended to find a solution to the requirement to improve the unit's use of alternative methods of communication that did not increase everyone's workload too much, and was interesting, this did not seem to be how his team had perceived his suggestion.

The relationship between the person or people instigating change and those required to change the way they work often affects the acceptance and implementation of new ways of working (Erwin and Garman 2010). Even when you are generally liked and respected by your colleagues, it may be expedient to ask yourself if there is anyone who you do not get on well with, or who feels threatened by you, how this might affect them accepting your ideas, and whether they have influence with other people. Rob was aware that whilst he generally got on well with his staff, some of them, especially those who had worked on the unit a long time, felt that he lacked practical experience or awareness of the realities of the job and the unit. Having reflected on how he had approached this issue, he felt that he had not really thought about involving the rest of the team in developing ideas for solutions. He now wanted to focus on hearing other people's thoughts about how the requirements of the review could be met. Although he had thought about how he might adapt his idea, he wanted to use the issue of communication to encourage the staff on the unit to think about their own practice, and that on the unit as a whole, and ways in which this might be developed. He particularly wanted to engage with the member of staff who spoke Makaton and British Sign Language, as she was well liked, respected, and had the advantage of having spent many years in the organisation. If she initiated, or supported, an idea for an innovation in communication, he felt others would follow. He also realised that unless she supported any proposed change, it might become a personal, if unstated, conflict between the two of them, which he wanted to avoid.

You may also have to consider how you will manage your ongoing motivation and ability to stay with your idea even when things do not go well, because the continued motivation of the person leading change influences whether or not a project reaches its goal (McPhee and Suryaparkash 2012). If you are a person who has no problem with sticking to a course of action against all odds, this may not be an issue, but it is probably expedient to consider whether your own response to and ability to manage opposition and setbacks will affect other people's engagement with change. Rob had initially thought that this change in practice would be relatively easy to effect. Now he was aware that it would be harder than he had anticipated, and wondered if he would be able to sustain his own motivation for carrying it through, particularly as he might not still be in post in two years time, when the next review took place. As a change leader, it can be useful to look not just at how you will support colleagues, but what support will be available to you (MacPhee and Suryaparkash 2012). By thinking in more depth about his own enthusiasm for the idea and what support he would need and have available, Rob felt able to make a realistic assessment of his own ability to commit to taking on a lead role in this change in practice.

Managing successful change requires you to consider how you will influence people's responses to an idea for innovation, and how you will sustain your own motivation.

Summary

Resistance to change can be positive, make you think through your plans diligently, and consider the possible pitfalls and difficulties as well as the advantages of what you plan to do. However, in order for change to happen, barriers to it often have to be overcome. These can include things that people openly state, and those that remain hidden. Amongst the most difficult barriers to overcome are apathy or silent resistance to change. When you are planning change, it is expedient to think about what the new way of working may mean for individuals and groups, what they are likely to see as the reasons for the request to change, what the potential benefits are, what individuals and groups stand to gain or lose, what effect the change will have on people's workloads in the short and long term, how the organisation and individuals within it have experienced change in the past, and how patient or client expectations will influence acceptance of any new way of working.

There is almost always likely to be some resistance to a change in practice, and although you need to think about this at the planning stage, it is equally important to keep track of it throughout the process of implementing a new way of working. Not all opposition will be immediately evident, and, as well as planning for known resistance to change, you need to remain alert to resistance developing as change is rolled out and progresses.

Key Points

Resistance to change can serve a positive purpose.

What people say they think about a plan for innovation may not reflect their actual views.

Change can create feelings of loss.

People's previous experiences of change can affect their acceptance of it.

Opposition by key individuals and groups influences the success of change.

Patients/clients can be key influences on whether or not change succeeds.

CASE STUDY

Tara works as a community nurse, and recently attended a study day where she heard about a new approach to dressing leg ulcer wounds, which seemed likely to be beneficial for some of her team's patients. She followed this up by finding out more information on the subject, and talking with the manufacturers. The evidence suggests that this approach would improve the outcomes for some patients, reduce the number of dressings that staff need to perform, and thus save them time and additional visits. Tara is now considering what the barriers to her idea becoming a reality may be.

How Might Individuals within the Team and the Team as a Whole Have Experienced Change in the Past?

The team that Tara works with have historically been relatively open to change, especially change initiated within the team. However, these changes have not always been sustained, and what seem to be good ideas have sometimes been used for a while, and then gradually abandoned, for no apparent reason. There have been at least two new ideas for leg ulcer dressings introduced in the past two years, both of which started well, but lost momentum. Several staff have now either become confused about what they are meant to be doing in terms of leg ulcer dressings, or tired of changes in what is recommended.

As a result, whilst the team are likely to be open to a suggestion from her, Tara thinks that there is a good chance that this will be seen as yet another idea about leg ulcer dressings, which will go nowhere. This may affect the team's enthusiasm to invest time in learning about it, and means that she needs to consider how she will convince her colleagues that this idea is not the latest in a series of fads about leg ulcer dressings.

What Other Changes Have the Team Experienced Recently?

The team that Tara works in have a new manager, which has led to some changes in role remits and responsibilities, and a new system of documentation being introduced. The team generally feel that they have not been consulted about these changes, and that they have been introduced in a manner that they do not like. The way changes have been implemented differs from how their previous manager worked, which was to consult frequently and in detail with the team before making any alterations to working practice.

Whilst Tara's idea does not emanate from the new manager, she thinks that there is a risk that this could be lost in the current distrust of change.

However, she also thinks that she may be able to use the current disapprobation for imposed change to her advantage, by adopting the 'bottom-up' approach to change which the team have traditionally used and favoured. Her aim is to present her idea, ask the team's views, and seek their support, in the way that new ideas were shared in the past.

What Evidence is There to Support This Change in Practice, and How Will Tara Present It?

Tara has collected a considerable amount of evidence to support her idea, including research, case reports, and explanations of the physiology behind how the new dressing works. However, she is aware that, because of the team's history of changes in leg ulcer dressings, this will need to be presented in a way that is compelling. She thinks that this will need to include not just why this dressing should be used, but how this change in practice will be sustained, and not become the third innovation that floundered.

Tara is planning to raise the issue of sustainability with her colleagues, because even if they do not voice this concern, she feels sure it will exist.

How Will This Change in Practice Affect Individual's Lives Outside of Work?

Tara does not think that this change in practice will affect people's personal lives. No extra work is required, and supplies are no more difficult to transport than the current dressings. It should in fact save time, and make workloads more manageable, as the dressings require changing less frequently than those currently in use. How May Established Routines or Practice Influence the Success of This Idea for Change?

The two recent attempts to change practice in relation to leg ulcer dressings mean that there is no established practice. Although this could make bringing a new protocol in easier, the recent history of change in relation to leg ulcer dressings might also mean that those who never really wanted to change their practice are even more reluctant to do so now.

What Losses Might Change Bring for Individuals or Groups?

The person who introduced the original change to leg ulcer dressings has now left the team, and the other change was made at the request of a general practitioner who was not a part of the team, so Tara feels that there should be no sense of loss from those whose ideas are being replaced by hers. Nonetheless, for those who never wanted to change the way of managing leg ulcer dressings, her idea may still represent loss, as the two previous unsuccessful changes may have enabled them to hope that nothing will ever really change.

Tara thinks that the team as a whole may be experiencing loss at present, because of the other changes that are happening. She plans to prevent her idea from becoming a part of this by introducing the idea in a form the team was previously familiar and comfortable with.

Will People Feel Confident about Their Ability to Work in the New Way?

Tara feels that confidence in the practicalities of using the new dressings will not be an issue for her team, as they are very easy to apply. However, her colleagues will need clarification on what to do if wounds do not respond as expected. As the dressings need changing less frequently than the ones currently in use they may also need assurance that they should not feel tempted to change the dressings more frequently than necessary.

How Will Individual and Group Views Affect Each Other?

There are several people in the team who are unhappy about the changes that had happened recently, and the opinions of two of them are strongly influential on overall team morale. If they see Tara's idea as just one more of the recent, and unwelcome, changes, it is likely that the whole team will be influenced by their views.

Will the Objections That People Have Be Openly Stated?

Tara is not sure that all possible objections to her idea will be openly stated. If anyone has an objection to the dressing in question, or questions about its efficacy, she is sure this will be stated, as the team is good at sharing new ideas and challenging one another to make sure that innovations are sensible before allowing them to proceed. It is also likely that she will have the chance to defend why yet another dressing is being recommended.

However, she feels that the underlying ethos of change fatigue and distrust may not be mentioned. She has decided that she will acknowledge that everyone had been experiencing a lot of change lately, to give an opening for anyone who wants to mention this to do so, and to provide herself with an opportunity to explain that her idea is not a part of this less popular approach to change.

Will Patients Influence whether or not Change Succeeds?

The new dressings will directly affect patients, some of whom are used to a particular dressing and may be reluctant to try something new. Tara is aware that patient views are likely to feed into staff views, and opposition by patients make it difficult, or impossible, for staff to use the new approach.

To counter this, she plans to ask each team to devise a list of patients who currently have leg ulcer wounds that they feel would be suitable for the new dressing, and identify which patients are likely to be willing to try this approach. She then plans to roll the new way of working out as a pilot, with patients who agreed to try this, so that those who are opposed to the idea do not become a barrier to change, and staff do not feel that they have to coerce patients to try a new approach.

An additional, and possibly unstated, barrier for some patients may be that the community nurses will visit them less often. Whilst for many nurses and patients this will be an advantage, for some patients it will mean that they lose a visit that they value. Tara feels that this needs to be acknowledged, and questions asked as to whether, in some cases, alternative social support should be considered, particularly where the nurse is a patient's only daily visitor.

Tara thinks that introducing the new dressing as a pilot will enable her to review the outcomes of using it, and then develop the implementation further following this (if appropriate). This may make it less likely that this change will, like its predecessors, last for a while, but slowly fade away, because the piloting process will mean it requires continued input, and the need for feedback will mean that staff and patients' views are obtained, as well as evidence of the effectiveness of the approach. The piloting process will provide Tara with a legitimate opportunity to give regular feedback to the team, and keep this initiative on everyone's agenda.

GUIDED WORK

This section revisits the learning outcomes covered in the chapter. You may want to complete it alone, or with colleagues.

1. Understand the potential value of resistance to change.

Think about a change in practice in your workplace where some objections to the innovation were raised (this may be recent or in the past).

- Did these hold change back?
- Did any of them have positive effects?

2. Recognise a range of possible causes of resistance to change.

Think about a change in practice in your workplace that encountered some resistance (this may be the same as the one you identified above).

- List the stated causes of this resistance.
- Consider whether there were likely to be any unstated, as well as stated, reasons for people resisting this innovation.

3. Consider how individual and group resistance to change can influence one another.

For the change you identified in 2, make a list of the individuals or groups who resisted change.

- Think about who they might have been influenced by.
- Think about who they might in turn have influenced.
- Identify whether the resistance of any individual or individuals affected how the team as a whole viewed the innovation.

4. Appreciate the significance of opinion leaders and key stakeholders in overcoming resistance to change.

Think of a change in practice that you have experienced (it may be one of the ones described above).

- Who were the key stakeholders?
- What was at stake for them?
- Who were the opinion leaders?
- Why did their opinion count?
- What were their views on the innovation?
- How did this affect the success or otherwise of the innovation?

5. Plan innovation in a manner that is likely to minimise resistance to it.

Identify a change in practice that you would be interested in making in your workplace. Consider what might be, or become, barriers to this happening, and how you could address them. You might include:

- Why this innovation is being suggested.
- The evidence you have to support this innovation.

- How individuals within the team, and the team as a whole, have experienced change in the past.
- Other recent or current changes.
- How this change in practice will affect individual's lives outside of work.
- How established routines or practice will be affected by this change.
- Losses that your idea might bring for individuals or groups.
- Whether people will feel confident about their ability to work in the new way.
- How individual and group views will affect each other.
- How patients/clients will influence whether or not this change is accepted.
- Whether the objections people may have will be openly stated or not.

Additional Resources

Barriers to change:
http://www.nice.org.uk/media/AF1/73/HowToGuideChangePractice.pdf   and
http://www.institute.nhs.uk/quality_and_service_improvement_tools/quality_
and_service_improvement_tools/human_dimensions_-_human_barriers_to_
change.html and http://www.york.ac.uk/res/e-society/projects/8/8briefingdoc.
pdf and http://www.nwacademy.nhs.uk/downloads/documents/microsite_ests/
e3_1722011_resistance_and_barriers_to_change.pdf

Change and loss:
http://ezinearticles.com/?Loss-And-Change&id=1195635

Resistance to change:
http://www.businessperform.com/change-management/resistance_to_change.
html

Successful implementation of change:
http://www.health.vic.gov.au/qualitycouncil/downloads/successfully_
implementing_change.pdf

6

Rolling Out New Practice

Chapter Learning Outcomes

After studying this chapter, the reader will be able to:

- Identify the right time to roll out an innovation in practice
- Understand measures that can be taken to maintain motivation for change during the early stages of implementation
- Consider how different levels of support and enthusiasm for change can be managed
- Develop strategies to manage problems or setbacks during the implementation of change.

Summary

This chapter focuses on the point at which planning for change is complete, and a new way of working is being rolled out. It discusses selecting the right time to initiate a new way of working; maintaining motivation whilst change is being implemented; concurrently managing different levels of support and enthusiasm; and managing problems, difficult situations, or setbacks.

Ben is the Team Leader of a community mental health team, which covers a large geographical area, and whose members are based in three offices. Four years ago the team moved to using electronic records. However, a number of staff, particularly those based in one office, still used paper records most of the time. The records system became fairly chaotic, with different methods of documentation being used in different areas and for different clients. Because of this, a decision was made to move to one new, electronic, system of record keeping. Ben has been involved in setting this up with the support of the IT department and three of his staff, one from each of the office bases.

They began designing the new approach in April and planned to roll it out on 1st November. By the end of October, Ben thought that this was still a realistic goal.

Knowing You Are Ready

The timing of the roll out of change in practice may sometimes be entirely date bound; for example, if there is an imposed deadline for implementation and no delay is permitted. However, if this is not the case, it is important to be sure that you are ready for the new way of working to be initiated, not just that the selected date has arrived.

It can be valuable to stick to dates, because there will always be something else you could do to prepare for a new way of working. In addition, as Chapter 5 identified, change can invoke feelings and responses similar to those associated with loss (Price 2008), and deferring the start date can feed into any degree of denial that the change will ever really go ahead. On the other hand, if things are not ready, rolling new practice out at a given point will certainly end in failure; it is therefore sensible to reschedule your launch date. If you do alter the date when change will be rolled out, it is expedient to select a time that you can definitely keep to, in order to avoid constant slippage. If the date for implementing change is repeatedly delayed, it is likely to reduce motivation amongst your supporters, and allow those who are hoping to avoid change to believe, and to convince others, that it will never actually happen.

If you have made a plan that includes everything that has to happen before change is rolled out, it will help you to know whether everything is ready, or whether there are still essential tasks to be achieved. Ben had planned to introduce the new system on 1st November, and, although there was no absolute obligation to use that day, everything that the action plan said should be done had been done. Most people seemed to accept, or be resigned to, the change in practice, and although two people still opposed it, he suspected that this would not change, regardless of what preparatory work was done. There was therefore nothing to be gained from further delays.

Choosing the right time to roll out change can be crucial to its success.

Having Everything in Place

A part of the immediate preparation for rolling out new practice is checking that the practicalities required are in place. This includes making sure that everything that is needed for the new way of working is available, and that there is enough of it (NICE 2007, Paton and McCalman 2008: 142–149). If all the practical requirements for a new system are not in place, it makes it too easy for anyone who wants to criticise or sabotage the innovation to do so, and makes it difficult for your supporters to defend the project. It is likely that a percentage of people will be fairly indifferent about any new way of working (Giangreco and Peccei 2005), and this group will probably follow the path of least resistance in terms of whether or not to adopt change. Making the new way of working the easiest option by having everything that is needed available, and ensuring that previous practice is difficult to continue with, increases the chance of those who are indifferent adopting the new system. Part of Ben's preparation was to check that everyone had access to the new system of documentation: that the links that took people to each type of documentation worked, and that all the computers that people used (both in offices and whilst they were out on their caseloads) could and automatically did access and use the new documentation. During the two weeks before the system was launched, he checked with each person in the team that they could access the system, and knew how to use it. On the day when the new way of working was rolled out Ben removed all the old paperwork from offices, and put reminders in the places where supplies had been about the new system. He did not want people to have the chance to forget to use the new approach, or to be able to deliberately use paper documentation. He also made sure that old links on the computer system were disabled, to stop people from using them. Ben's intention was to make using the new system the obvious and easy option, and to make it difficult to do otherwise.

One of Ben's aims was to ensure that, on the day that the new system was rolled out, everything was in place for it, and that the message was very clear that the new way of working was irretrievably here. He was especially aware that the group who had effectively avoided changing the way they worked when electronic documentation was first introduced might think that this could happen again. He wanted to clarify, in a non-confrontational manner, that it could not.

As well as checking the technical and practical aspects of change, it is useful to make sure that anyone who said they would do something towards the new way of working still will, and has remembered that now is the time to do it. Ben's preparations included checking that the member of staff from the IT department who had said that he would be available in the first week of the new records being used to troubleshoot any problems was still available. Similarly, he checked with the three people who had agreed to act as the change champions for their office bases (those promoting the new way of working and encouraging their colleagues to use it; Scott et al. 2003, Soo et al. 2009) that they were still on board for the roll out day.

Having all the practicalities in place makes it easier for people who want to change to do so, and harder for those who want to sabotage an innovation to succeed.

Checklist for Rolling Out Change

Is this when you had planned to roll out the new way of working?
Have all the preparations been made?
Are all the necessary resources available?
Are all your key support systems/people still available?
Has any training that was needed taken place?
Are enough people on board to make success possible?

Maintaining Motivation

Like all other aspects of change management, the people aspects of rolling out change are often the most demanding. One of the challenges of introducing new practice is not just to get the new way of working in place, but to maintain and develop people's motivation for doing things in the new way once it has been set up. Maintaining motivation in the long term is explored in Chapter 9, but maintaining motivation through the early days of a new way of working is important: if everyone has given up on the new system by day five, then thoughts of long-term maintenance become superfluous.

Previous chapters have outlined the importance of involving people in change, and valuing their contributions, views, and ideas. This remains important once the new way of working is in progress, so that they still feel involved, up to date with what is happening, and valued (Giangreco and Peccei 2005, Hall and Hord 2011: 150–151). In the early days of rolling out the new system of record keeping, Ben contacted his colleagues who were acting as the change champions in the three office bases and his colleague in the IT department on a regular basis. He kept them up to date with where the project was at, advised them of any developments or problems encountered, asked for feedback on the system, and thanked them for their ongoing support. He wanted to make them feel that he still valued their involvement, needed them on board, and that they remained a part of a project team, with an important role to play. By visiting the three bases that his team worked from regularly, Ben was able to thank people for the efforts they were making to use the new system, and give feedback where appropriate.

Communication has been identified as a vital part of achieving successful change (Jimmieson et al. 2008). When new practice is rolled out, as well as keeping your core team on board, a steady stream of communication with everyone involved is vital. This can help people to become confident in the new system and those running it if they were not already, and if they were, it maintains and develops that confidence (Giangreco and Peccei 2005, Hall and Hord 2011: 150–152). To this end, Ben developed a strategy to keep in close contact with his staff over the first week of the new system being rolled out in order to hear their views, respond to any issues that arose, and let them know how things were going with the new approach to documentation.

Stay in Touch When Change Is Rolled Out . . .

To remind everyone about what is happening
To maintain enthusiasm amongst your supporters
To make those who are making an effort feel valued
To demonstrate that you are engaged with the roll out
To hear how things are going and act on this

Maintaining communication with those who are involved in working in a new way means that you are likely to get feedback on how things are going, hear about positive events or influences, any problems or challenges that are arising behind the scenes, and pick up on any undercurrents of disengagement or opposition (Giangreco and Peccei 2005, Hall and Hord 2011: 145). Because of the nature of his team's work, and the diverse locations they covered, Ben did not always see them as regularly as he would have liked to. They had weekly meetings, but not everyone attended them. By making himself available, staying in touch with his change champions, and visiting his team's bases regularly during the early days of the new system, he intended to pick up on any problems, aspects of the system that needed changing, and be seen to be present, and interested. He hoped that this would also enable him to see how things were really going, rather than just what was reported.

Ben wanted to keep the new way of working front central, so that people knew it was not forgotten and did not forget about it (Hall and Hord 2011: 150–151). By visiting and communicating with his team regularly he planned to be able to give informal updates on the success of the project so far, and in this way keep them focused on continuing to use the new documentation. He scheduled a slot to feed back on the new records system at the weekly team meetings for the first two months after it was introduced, then every second meeting, then monthly until the final evaluation at six months. He wanted to keep the new way of working on the agenda of the meetings, but decrease the frequency of discussions about it as the formal evaluation date approached to see if it really had become embedded in day-to-day practice without regular reminders. He also thought that by gradually reducing the frequency of feedback he would move people away from the idea that the system was new, to the concept of it being standard practice.

Communicating clearly and consistently when change is rolled out increases the chance of the innovation being successful.

Managing Problems

People's acceptance of change is likely to be increased if things appear to be going reasonably well in the early days of its implementation, but how you manage any problem that occurs at this time are equally, or even more, important in gaining and maintaining the support of your colleagues. This includes concerns being listened to and acted on, being seen to collaborate with others in finding solutions to problems, and progress in resolving difficulties being evident and reported on (Reed and Turner 2005, Hall and Hord 2011: 115). Those who are working with a new system day-to-day may know things about it that you do not, and if something is a concern to one person, it may be to others as well. In addition, if you are not seen to be listening to and acting on concerns, then the person or persons involved may not feel that they and their opinion are valued, cease to support you, and use this as ammunition to encourage others not to do so (Cameron and Green 2009: 124, Hall and Hord 2011: 150–151).

Although listening to, believing, and acting on individual concerns is important, it is also useful to think about the cause of any apparent problem, and to look for patterns, or common themes, related to problems that arise (Hall and Hord 2011: 180). Chapter 2 described the need to take some time to analyse any problem in practice that creates a need for change, and similarly looking into what the real problems or issues are when change is being implemented is expedient. Looking at the cause of any concerns makes it more likely that you will find an appropriate solution to the problem itself, rather than managing its effect. You may also find that more than one complaint or concern has the same root cause, and by identifying this, it may be possible to effect a solution that addresses more than one issue (van Meijel et al. 2004).

On the second day of the new records being introduced, Ben found one member of staff who was still using paper records because she claimed that the link to the new system was not working on her computer. Ben worked with her on this and found the link working perfectly. Discussing the issue with her, and then going through the new process on the computer alongside her, alerted Ben to the possibility that this person (who worked in the area where paper records had still been used) was probably looking for reasons to avoid using the new documentation, and might be inclined to dissuade others as well. As he had deliberately removed all the paper documents from the offices, he politely asked her where she had found them, ostensibly so as to avoid future confusion. The answer was not very clear, but he felt that he had identified a possible source of resistance, and had made clear that he was available, willing to provide additional input and troubleshooting, but also monitoring the situation and likely to pick up on problems. In this way Ben provided coaching in the new process, addressed the person's stated concerns, but also made clear that the change was here to stay, and worked on reducing any sabotage of the new system that the individual in question might create (Hall and Hord 2011: 150–151). Another person from the same office advised Ben that they could not access the new system on their laptop when they were out on caseload work, and that their team felt that they should use paper records whilst out on visits, and record these electronically when they returned to base. However, when Ben explored the problem it was difficult to identify why accessing the electronic system had been problematic. He suspected that these two apparently different problems stemmed from the same desire to retain paper copies of the records. Whilst one apparently related to a desktop computer and one to a laptop, the issue appeared to Ben to be the same: this particular office was not really signed up to the new way of working, and he would have to continue to work closely with them to embed the electronic records system.

Being seen to listen to concerns and manage any problems or challenges is as important as highlighting the positive aspects of change.

Managing Differing Levels of Support

To successfully roll out new practice you generally need a critical mass who have bought into it and are ready to work in the new way (Cameron and Green 2009: 185, Hall and Hord 2011: 223). If you do not have enough people on board then it is unlikely that your change will work. However, the balance between waiting too long and waiting until you have enough support can be a fine one. Ben was aware that two staff in one office still did not accept the new approach to record keeping, but suspected that until it was introduced and became inevitable they would not accept it however much he worked with them. Although a few dissatisfied individuals can cause great problems (Scott et al. 2003), whilst you are working hard with a few stragglers, and waiting for them to come on board, those who were enthusiastic may lose interest. One of the challenges involved in managing change is that whilst some people will be, and will continue to be, very enthusiastic from the outset, others will not be, and will take some time to come on board (Hall and Hord 2011: 119–124). The key to managing differing levels of support is to try to gauge where different people are at, and to give them input and tasks appropriate to that stage (Golden 2006). Keeping those on board who have always been there, being aware of those who may be wavering, and knowing who is likely to influence them, whilst at the same time trying to increase the number of your supporters and the strength of their support is part of the juggling process of managing change (Golden 2006).

The usual pattern of people adopting change is sometimes represented by an s shaped curve, where support for innovation starts slowly, gradually picks up speed, then flattens off, with a final few coming on board at the very end of the process (Hall and Hord 2011: 223). In any process of change, there are likely to be innovators, who initiate the change or are keen for it to take place, and early adopters, who agree with the idea for change and create the impetus required to carry it forward. These groups, who essentially lead the change, are often followed by what are known as the early majority: who adopt change to fall into place as they see others accepting it, and the late majority, who initially reject the change, but eventually conform when everyone else seems to be doing so. The final group are the laggards, who continue to reject change, forever or until the new way of doing things becomes established practice (Rogers 1995, Hall and Hord 2011: 220–221). By the time you roll out change, the innovators will be established as leaders or champions of change, and the early adopters will have accepted the plan and been ready to do things in the new way for some time. The early majority are likely to have been on board, even if not as committed as some, for a while, and the late majority will probably be just about ready to work in the new way, but still wavering. The laggards will not yet be ready to adopt the new way of working.

Individuals who are at different stages in adopting change are likely to influence each other. Your intention should be to make this work to your advantage, for example, by harnessing the commitment of those who have embraced change to bring others on board, rather than allowing the laggards to undercut adoption by others and derail to process of change (Hall and Hord 2011: 221–222). There had been few real enthusiasts for the new record keeping system. Ben and one other person who felt strongly about introducing the new record keeping system because of the difficulties they had encountered with working with at least two different approaches had shared much of the work of developing and introducing the new system. They had been the innovators, and the main agents of change. Ben's colleague in the IT department had also been quite enthusiastic about the project, and there had been a small group of early adopters amongst the team, two of whom had become the change champions for their offices. However, a large percentage of people came on board as the early majority or late majority when it was clear that most people were not objecting, or that the change would happen. They were those who were most likely to be persuaded by the laggards to abandon the new way of working, because they did not really care a great deal whether the electronic records system happened or not.

Ben thought that knowing who still did not really want to work in the new way, and those who were most likely to be influenced by them, would help him to minimise their influence and to target the people whose support he would probably have to work hardest on maintaining. He was aware that the group that had previously managed to resist moving to electronic records had, in general, been the most resistant to this project and was the only office with people who still really opposed the idea of electronic records. He knew that those who now accepted the idea but worked in this area were the most likely to be persuaded that it was, in fact, unnecessary and could be ignored. For this reason, he visited that group more frequently than others in the early days of the new way of working, addressed the continued use of paper records, and opposed their suggestion of using paper records whilst out on visits. He wanted to clarify that ignoring the new records system would not be possible on this occasion, and to openly build on and show that he valued the support that the new system did have in that office.

At the same time, Ben wanted to avoid becoming so preoccupied with two resisters, who might never support the new way of working however much effort he made, that he lost sight of those who were wavering or needed supportive input to keep them on board (Hall and Hord 2011: 74). The detractors were the minority, and whilst they could still sabotage the process of change, he wanted to keep them in perspective. He made sure that he also visited and remained in contact with the areas where there were no known problems, and with his change champions, to ensure that whilst he was focusing on the laggards, the rest of the process had not quietly failed.

You may have to accept that some people will never adopt a new way of working (Rogers 1995, Hall and Hord 2011: 220–221). Nonetheless, it is important to avoid creating an environment in which to ever come on board would be too big a climb down for anyone. When Ben found people opposing the use of the new electronic records, overtly or covertly, he avoided confrontation, but instead invited them to explore the difficulties with him, helped them to solve the problem they presented to him, and often asked if they would be happy to feed back this solution to any other team members who encountered it. As well as wanting to maintain goodwill, his intention was to create a situation in which if and when they were ready to adopt the new way of working, they could see it, and present it to others, as the problems they had had with the system having been ironed out, not a battle that they had lost.

People will accept change at different rates: a few will usually be enthusiastic from the start, and one or two never really come on board. The majority will go with the path of least resistance, or the most influential sources of opinion.

Recalling Your Aims

When you roll out change, keeping your original aim and objectives in mind is important for you, and for those who are working with you. Sometimes all your attention is focused on the procedure and process of a new way of working, and rightly so because you want things to go well, but at the same time you do not want to get into a situation where the aim is lost in its achievement. It is likely that as you roll out change and implement it, you will have to make alterations to how you thought things would work, and what you thought you would do. If you keep your original aim clearly in mind, you can decide if the deviations you make will take you too far off track (Golden 2006).

The primary aim of the new record keeping system was that Ben's team would all use the same documentation, and that this would be done electronically. Although he and his two key colleagues and change champions had spent some time in devising and piloting assessment tools and ongoing documentation, there was no real problem with tweaking these, redesigning them, and adjusting them, provided that the core aim of using one, electronic, system was achieved. On one occasion, Ben found that a member of staff had started to use paper records alongside the electronic system because she did not feel that the electronic version allowed her to effectively record the events from a recent case conference that her client had been involved in. A decision had been made by all concerned to discontinue using the form in question, because it was felt that the information could be better recorded within the core electronic documentation. Nevertheless, Ben said that if the team as a whole felt that it was important that this form still existed, he could arrange for it be made available, completed and stored electronically. This form itself was not really the issue, and Ben wanted to avoid the core aim of the project being lost in discussion of one form, whose value was not central to the decision to use electronic records. Instead, he used it as an opportunity to show that he was open to ideas and suggestions, and that he was happy to make changes in light of feedback, provided that the core aim of using one system of electronic record keeping was still met.

Being clear about the aim of an innovation makes it possible to identify what concessions you can make without sacrificing your goal.

Summary

The process of rolling out new practice is a vital part of any change initiative: unless it happens, nothing changes, and how it is carried out affects whether or not the new way of working is adopted (Paton and McCalman 2008: 144). The process of rolling out change includes putting in place the practicalities required, but also using appropriate strategies and communication to maintain motivation and retain existing support, whilst concurrently managing different levels of support and enthusiasm within the team concerned. It is also important to keep focused on the original aim of the new way of working as change is rolled out, so as to stay true to this, despite any adjustments that may become necessary.

Key Points

Choosing the right time to roll out new practice can be critical to its success.

Checking that the key resources and systems are still available at the point of rolling out change is vital.

Maintaining people's motivation in the early days of an innovation being implemented is crucial.

When change is rolled out, people within a team are likely to still have different levels of support and enthusiasm for it.

Managing problems, difficult situations, or setbacks effectively is as important as highlighting positive aspects of change.

CASE STUDY

Amy works in an accident and emergency (A&E) department. Difficulties were reported between A&E and some of the wards related to patients being transferred, and, because of this, a new protocol for transferring patients from A&E to wards and departments has been drawn up, piloted, and is now being introduced.

The aim of the protocol is to ensure clear communication regarding the transfer of patients from A&E to wards and departments.

The objectives of the protocol are

- One person from A&E will liaise with the ward or department concerned, and co-ordinate the transfer of each patient.
- An agreed level of information on the patient and their condition will be provided as a minimum.
- A timeframe for transfer will be decided on and adhered to.
- Any disagreements over transfer will be referred through the senior nurse on call (bleep holder) for the specialty in question.
- The receiving ward or department will be advised when the patient is leaving A&E.

There were mixed feelings within A&E about the new protocol: some people considered it cumbersome and an unnecessary replacement for something that generally worked well, some thought that it was an overreaction to unfounded grumbling, others considered it useful because it clarified what could reasonably be expected from each party, and where disagreements should be directed.

Amy was a part of the team who developed the protocol, and as such is also involved in rolling it out.

How Did the Team Decide that This Was the Right Time to Roll Out the New Way of Working?

The plan was to develop the protocol, pilot this for four weeks, evaluate it, make any necessary adjustments, and then roll the protocol out within two weeks if the pilot indicated that this was appropriate. The pilot was complete, a few minor adjustments and additions had been made, and two weeks after the pilot there was no more to be done, so the time seemed right to roll the protocol out.

Were the Necessary Practicalities in Place?

Copies of the protocol had been laminated, and placed by the telephones in A&E to remind staff of it when they contacted wards.

The Protocol Had Been Placed in the Unit Procedure Book

Staff had been advised that the new protocol was now in use by means of email, the unit communication book, information placed on the unit notice boards, and department meetings.

The protocol had been agreed with change champions in each ward and department, and protocols issued to these areas, including laminated copies for display by telephones. The dissemination and implementation at ward and department level rested largely with the change champions, but Amy and her team had also visited these areas, to check that the protocols had been received, were displayed, and known about.

The change champions on the wards and departments and senior nurses who co-ordinated the bleep holding rota were reminded that the new protocol was being rolled out a week before the event, and on the day itself.

What Was Done to Maintain the Motivation of Those Who Supported the Project?

Amy was one of a team of four people involved in developing the new protocol. The team's motivation had been maintained during piloting by them being involved in gathering evaluative data on the new system, and meeting weekly to discuss what seemed to be good about the system and what changes might need to be made.

Once the new way of working was rolled out, the team had an evaluation strategy that involved formal evaluation at two months, six months, and a year after implementation. The core team thus remained involved. They also planned to work on a conference paper about the new protocol.

Those who supported the innovation but who were not on the planning team also needed to be kept on board, especially as there was some opposition to the new protocol, which could easily discourage them from continuing to favour it. The planning team gave regular feedback on the positive aspects of the project, and where particular feedback from wards, staff, patients or relatives was received, this was mentioned. For the first month, this feedback was being provided via a weekly email, at team meetings, and by written comments in the communication book. After this, monthly updates were to be provided, including findings from the formal evaluations at two months, six months, and a year. The intention of this ongoing feedback was to show how the protocol made a difference to patient care and working relations. After the initial weekly feedbacks, the frequency of reporting was to be decreased so as to avoid information overload. Change champions for the wards and departments were also a part of this communication network, and encouraged to feed back to their colleagues.

On a personal level, in the early days of implementation, staff who were seen to be using the new protocol were commended for this. Any particular positive feedback from the use of the protocol was reported to those concerned. The intention of this strategy was to serve both as a reinforcement of the value of this way of working to individuals, and as a reminder that the use of the new protocol was being noted. Any difficulties that arose were addressed with individuals at the time, and solutions explored, insti-gated, shared with the unit team and, if relevant, the wards or departments involved, so that problems and concerns were seen to be taken seriously and acted on.

What Was Done to Recruit Additional Support?

When the project was rolled out, there were a range of degrees of support for it. Recruiting additional support was achieved in a similar way to retaining the support of those who were on board, with the additional intention of convincing those who were wavering or unwilling to accept the new pro-tocol that it was here to stay, although it was possible to make reasonable adjustments to improve it. If people raised queries or made comments, they were invited to explore solutions with the team, so that they felt listened to, but were also encouraged to be a part of, and own, the solutions.

How Were Different Levels of Enthusiasm for the Project Managed?

Those who were the most enthusiastic about developing the protocol at the outset were in the core team (the initiators and early adopters). Those who became enthusiastic during the process of its development (the early major-ity) were often asked to take on specific roles, for example, linking with a ward or department, aiding in gathering evaluation data, or championing change on their shifts within the area they were working in.

At the same time as encouraging enthusiasm, the team were aware that an overemphasis on the project might be counterproductive. A balance was sought between asking people to participate and providing information, and constant discussion creating boredom with the subject. It was also important to see those detracting from the project within the greater picture of those who needed input to be kept on board. Two or three staff were strongly opposed to using the protocol, and seemed likely to remain so regardless of what happened. The team recognised that a great deal of time and effort, which could usefully be employed elsewhere, might be expended in attempt-ing to persuade them to comply, to little effect. Instead, they focused on developing and maintaining the enthusiasm of others, so as to overcome or lessen the impact of the two or three main detractors.

How Were Problems or Setbacks Managed?

If a problem with the protocol was reported, exploration with those who had noted it of exactly what that problem was, why it was thought to be a problem, its possible cause or causes, and what might be able to be done to resolve it was the approach that the team took. Outcomes and decisions were fed back to the individuals or wards/departments concerned, and included in the regular updates to all staff.

The intention of these steps was to ensure that people felt that their concerns were listened to and acted on; the causes rather than effects of problems were the focus of interventions; individuals were actively involved in the process of refining the protocol; and everyone was kept updated on how difficulties were being managed.

Whilst wanting to be seen to be responsive to feedback, the team were aware that constant tweaking and changing of the new protocol could be problematic. Therefore, unless there was an urgent need to do so, changes were generally scheduled to be made at the predetermined evaluation points of two months, six months and a year after introduction of the protocol. These milestones were shared with the unit as whole, so that it was known that there would sometimes be delays in changes to the protocol being effected.

Was There any Change from the Original Plan and, if so, Did This Detract from the Main Aim of the Project?

During the piloting phase, some minor changes to the protocol were made, however these did not detract from the aim of ensuring clear communication about patient transfers from A&E to wards and departments. Some of the changes improved on the original protocol. For example, an alteration to the proforma of what information would be provided improved the standard level of information on the patient's condition, and made communication clearer.

GUIDED WORK

This section revisits the learning outcomes covered in the chapter. You may want to complete it alone, or with colleagues.

1. Identify the right time to roll out an innovation in practice.

Think about a change in practice that you have been involved with or have seen being implemented. Do you know why it was implemented when it was? You could consider:

- Was there a requirement to implement it at any given time?
- Were all the necessary resources in place?

- Were the necessary practicalities were in place?
- Did enough people seem to support the idea?
- Did any key people oppose it?
- How might these factors have contributed to the innovation's success (or otherwise)?

2. Understand measures that can be taken to maintain motivation for change during the early stages of implementation.

For the change you identified above, reflect on what happened during the early days of this innovation:

- Were people kept up to date with what was happening?
- Were those leading or facilitating the innovation 'visible' at this time?
- Was feedback given on how things were going?
- Were people thanked or rewarded for the effort they were making?
- Were any practical difficulties acknowledged and dealt with?
- What effect did these measures have on the success (or otherwise) of the innovation?

3. Consider how different levels of support and enthusiasm for change can be managed.

For the innovation that you identified above:

- List the people who you recall being involved in or affected by it.
- Were these people the innovators, early adopters, early majority, late majority, or laggards?
- Was there any movement in which groups people belonged to as the change was implemented?
- What was done to keep those who supported the innovation on board?
- What was done to recruit more support from those who were wavering or opposed the innovation?
- How did this affect the success or otherwise of the innovation?

4. Develop strategies to manage problems or setbacks during the implementation of change.

For the change you have identified, think abut whether any problems or setbacks occurred during its implementation.

- How were these handled?
- Did this aid or hinder the success of the innovation?

Additional Resources

Resources on implementing change:
http://www.health.vic.gov.au/qualitycouncil/downloads/successfully_
implementing_change.pdf   and   http://www.lindsay-sherwin.co.uk/guide_
managing_change/html_implementing_change/0_implementing_change.htm

7

Multidisciplinary Change

Chapter Learning Outcomes

After studying this chapter, the reader will be able to:

- Distinguish multidisciplinary, interdisciplinary, and transdisciplinary working
- Identify whether more than one discipline needs to be involved in a given innovation
- Decide which individuals from different disciplines should take on key roles in change
- Appreciate the potential complexity of managing individual and group agendas and concerns in planning and implementing change.

Summary

This chapter discusses planning multidisciplinary change. It begins by distinguishing concepts of multidisciplinary, interdisciplinary, and transdisciplinary working and explores why these distinctions matter in change management. It then describes the process of identifying whether the involvement of more than one discipline in a proposed change is necessary; deciding which groups should be involved; deciding the level and type of input that will be required of them; identifying key players in each discipline; and identifying the potential complexity of managing individual and group agendas and concerns, whilst also keeping a focus on the primary aim of an innovation.

Alison is the pain nurse specialist for a surgical unit that comprises six wards: ENT surgery, general surgery, ophthalmic surgery, gynaecology, urology, and orthopaedics. The unit has a pain assessment tool that has been in use for many years, and a protocol for managing pain, which is also somewhat dated. Alison and Charlotte (an anaesthetist who has a special interest in pain management) want to develop a new protocol for assessing and managing post-operative pain. One of the challenges they face in developing this is the number of wards and departments that will need to be involved, and the range of professions and disciplines within these whose input will be needed.

What Type of Team Are You Dealing with?

Healthcare increasingly requires different professions and disciplines to work together (Royal College of Nursing and Royal College of Physicians 2006, Atwal and Jones 2007, MacPhee and Suryaparkash 2012). As a result, any change that takes place in healthcare is likely to involve a number of different disciplines. Although the principles of change management remain fairly constant, there are some specific considerations when the change being planned involves more than one profession or discipline.

Firstly, it is useful to think about exactly how the disciplines that are going to be involved in a change in practice work together: for example, the degree of collaboration, co-operation, and shared understanding that they have in their work. The most commonly differentiated terms related to disciplines working in association with one another are multidisciplinary, interdisciplinary, and transdisciplinary working (Choi and Pak 2006). These terms are not always clearly defined, and are often used interchangeably, although they do not refer to exactly the same concept (Choi and Pak 2006). Multidisciplinary working requires more than two healthcare staff, from different disciplines, to be involved in an individual's care (Wilson and Pirrie 2000). However, it generally focuses on disciplines with separate but interrelated functions and roles, who do not really alter their pre-existing discipline-based boundaries (Choi and Pak 2006, O'Neill and Cowman 2007, Korner 2010). Interdisciplinary working, in contrast, usually refers to situations where the roles and perspectives of different disciplines are integrated, and disciplinary boundaries blurred: staff may surrender some aspects of their traditional discipline-based role, and take on some of those of others (Choi and Pak 2006, O'Neill and Cowman 2007, Peng et al. 2008, Korner 2010). Transdisciplinary working takes the blurring of roles and boundaries seen in interdisciplinary working further, with these being transcended to the extent that the original disciplinary basis of each individual in the team cannot be distinguished in their day-to-day work (Choi and Pak 2006). The terms multidisciplinary, interdisciplinary, and transdisciplinary working are not the only ones used to describe how professions may work together, and are not always used in exactly these ways. However, they illustrate the principle that people who work in situations that involve more than one discipline may work together in very different manners. In terms of change management, how any team that involves different disciplines functions is likely to affect how changing that team's practice will best be managed.

Alison and Charlotte considered that they were dealing with a multidisciplinary, rather than interdisciplinary, or transdisciplinary team. There were occasional areas of role overlap within the team; for example, some activities were interchangeably performed by theatre nurses and operating department practitioners (ODPs). However, the general approach to care was that different disciplines carried out different, albeit complimentary and sometimes slightly overlapping, roles and functions. Whilst the staff that used the new protocol would all be involved in pain assessment and management, with the shared goal of ensuring that patients were, as far as possible, pain free, they would not be carrying out the same functions. They might also not have completely shared priorities, goals, and values related to pain management.

When you are managing change in a team that includes different disciplines, it can be useful to think about whether or not your aim or objectives include altering the way the team functions. For instance, whether you intend to change an aspect of practice that affects the whole team but retains their existing approach to collaborative working, or to bring about change in a way that alters the way the team members work together as well as addressing the subject in question. In the long term, Alison and Charlotte were interested in developing approaches to pain management that adopted a more interdisciplinary approach. However, whilst they both thought that it might be possible to use the protocol development process as a step towards exploring the potential for this, it was not the main focus of their current work. Their priority was to develop a jointly agreed and workable pain management protocol that all disciplines would use.

Thinking about the way in which different disciplines within a team work together can help you to decide how to approach change.

Having decided what type of team is going to be involved in and affected by a change in practice, it is useful to consider what will be gained by involving the different disciplines concerned in planning change.

How Disciplines Might Work Together

Multidisciplinary: disciplines with separate functions and roles work together but do not change their existing role boundaries.

Interdisciplinary: the roles, perspectives, and boundaries of different disciplines are blurred.

How Disciplines Might Work Together   *continued*

Transdisciplinary: disciplinary roles and boundaries are transcended and individuals' original disciplinary background cannot be distinguished in their day-to-day work.

Why Involve the Multidisciplinary Team in Planning Change?

Involving representatives from across the disciplines, which will be involved in a change in practice at the planning stage, is important because although all healthcare staff theoretically subscribe to the same broad goals, their priorities, professional cultures, beliefs, and values may be different (Scott et al. 2003, Parkin 2009: 115). In addition to profession- or discipline-specific values, values may differ between groups or specialities within one profession (Scott et al. 2003, Reinhardt and Keller 2009). For example, the views of and priority afforded to pain management might differ between surgeons and anaesthetists, and mean that their views on any new way of working related to pain management were not exactly the same. Charlotte and Alison also thought that whilst some disciplines would welcome protocols for pain assessment and management, others might see them as impinging on their professional judgment or freedom. Involving representatives from all the disciplines that would use the new protocol in its development would provide the opportunity to discuss such issues, and determine how best to address them.

Including all the disciplines who will ultimately need to work in a new way in its planning can enable them to appreciate the skills each one can contribute, or need to develop, in order for the innovation to be effective (Ross et al. 2005). This can include their commonalities and differences in expertise, knowledge, education, and regulatory requirements (Royal College of Nursing and Royal College of Physicians 2006). In devising a new pain management protocol, assumptions might exist about what the different disciplines knew or did not know, what they could or could not do, what their day-to-day workload and way of working was, and what their permissible professional boundaries were. This might include issues such as who could and could not set up or change epidural analgesia, as well as why this was. Each discipline knowing this type of information about their colleagues would mean that when the protocol was developed, not only would the required actions be clear, but why certain boundaries or regulations existed would also be known.

The practical implications of a new protocol, as well as their potentially differing values and professional regulations, were likely to be different for each discipline. Whilst Alison and Charlotte took lead roles in pain management, they did not necessarily know the minutiae of how the day-to-day processes involved in assessing and managing pain worked in practice for each discipline. If the disciplines involved worked together on the development of the new protocol, the outcome was more likely to be usable and acceptable to them all (Ross et al. 2004, Hall and Hord 2011: 148).

One intention of involving all the disciplines concerned in developing the new protocol was to make it something that would work for everyone who would need to use it, whilst another was to address some of the people factors involved in change. Assessing individual readiness for change and working to get a critical mass who support a new way of working is important in any change, as discussed in Chapters 4 and 6 (Holt et al. 2007, Cameron and Green 2009: 185, Hall and Hord 2011: 219–224, Pare et al. 2011). When the change concerned involves a team that includes various disciplines from different wards and departments, planning has to take into account how ready all of these groups, as well as the individuals within them, are for change (Saull-McCaig et al. 2006). This would almost certainly be an unachievable task for one or two people. By engaging representatives from all the relevant disciplines in their core planning team, Alison and Charlotte hoped that they would have people who could work closely with the individuals and teams who would use the new protocol. These people would be better placed than them to assess the readiness for change, driving and restraining forces, and the barriers to change described in Chapters 3–6 within each discipline and ward or department. Knowing these, and being able to take them into account in planning how and when to implement change would increase the likelihood that the new way if working would be successful.

Involving Different Disciplines in Planning Change Means

More perspectives are heard.
The benefits and challenges for each discipline can be identified.
Discipline-specific knowledge, skills, and boundaries can be understood.
Change champions for each discipline can be identified.
Key representatives from each team involved own the innovation.

How and by whom information about a new way of working is presented to those who will be affected by it is likely to affect its success, and sometimes information is better received if it is provided by a member of the discipline in question. Those from within a discipline may better understand the cultural and practical issues which a new way of working will present for their colleagues, and be seen to have more credibility than an outsider (Golden 2006). It was likely to be important for nurses to be told about the new protocol for pain management by someone who would be viewed as understanding the day-to-day practicalities of how it would work and fit with their other work and documentation. This would probably be best achieved by the information being delivered by another nurse who was based in the same or a similar clinical area. People from the discipline or area concerned are also more likely than others to know what the important points for the group they work with are, their culture and history of change, and what may influence their response to change in general, or this change in particular (McCabe 2010).

As change is rolled out, it is usually important to have change champions, who can work alongside those required to work in the new way on a day-to-day basis (Saull-McCaig et al. 2006, Reinhardt and Keller 2009). In multidisciplinary change management, and particularly where change needs to be effected across more than one ward or department, it is very valuable to have change champions from every discipline or department involved. If all the disciplines that will be involved in a new way of working are represented at the planning stage, then you probably have an automatic supply of change champions.

If an innovation will require more than one discipline to change the way they work, people from those disciplines need to be involved at the planning stage.

It was clear that it would be beneficial for Alison and Charlotte to involve a number of disciplines in planning and developing the new protocol. The next step was to determine exactly which disciplines this would mean, and who should represent them.

Deciding Which Groups Need to Be Involved in Planning Change

Mapping out which disciplines will be affected by a change in practice is a good way to decide which ones need to be involved in planning a new way of working (Scott et al. 2003). If you realise after you have rolled out change that a group was omitted from the planning, you may have already alienated them, or missed out an important point that only they would know about and which will derail the new way of working. When Alison and Charlotte thought about who they would need to have on the planning group for the pain management protocol, they thought through the patient pathway from theatre, to ward, to discharge, so as to make sure that no stages were missed out, and that who would be involved in using the new protocol at each point was identified. They identified that the protocol would essentially involve two elements of pain management: pain assessment, and the prescription and administration of drugs.

Post-operative pain assessment was mainly carried out by nurses, although medical staff and physiotherapists also contributed to it. For this part of the protocol, it was therefore appropriate to include nurses (on the wards and in the recovery area), surgeons, anaesthetists, and physiotherapists. In relation to the prescription and drug administration element of the protocol, prescription was primarily the responsibility of anaesthetists, surgeons, and pharmacists. Administration of medication was almost always the responsibility of nurses. However, because part of the protocol would also deal with infused analgesia, and first doses given in theatre, theatre nurses and ODPs would also be involved. Technicians would be affected as well because they were responsible for the central availability and maintenance of infusion pumps, and troubleshooting problems that arose during pump use. For this part of the protocol, pharmacists, anaesthetists, surgeons, nurses, ODPs, and technicians therefore needed to be involved. The list of the disciplines to be involved in the development of the pain management protocol for the surgical unit therefore included anaesthetists; surgeons; pharmacists; ODPs; nurses from the wards, recovery area, and theatres; physiotherapists; and medical technicians.

As well as deciding which disciplines to involve in planning change, it is necessary to decide which grades of staff from each discipline, and how many of each, should be involved. Alison and Charlotte thought that the surgeons and anaesthetists should be represented by consultant grade staff as they were the most constant presence in wards and departments. In addition, unequal power and status can be a barrier to change (Reinhardt and Keller 2009), and consultants were seen as those most likely to be in a position to endorse prescribing trends and actions to be taken by medical staff. Whilst the intention was not to use a power coercive approach to change management (Chin and Benne 1985), they thought that it would be important for those who had authority and influence over junior staff to be signed up to the new way of working.

Six surgical specialities would be involved in using the new protocol, but it was thought that to have a consultant surgeon representative from each of these would be excessive in terms of keeping the planning group to a manageable size. Charlotte discussed with the surgeons and anaesthetists who should be involved: two surgeons were chosen to represent all their colleagues and one additional anaesthetist was taken on board. This gave a total of four medical staff on the working group.

In nursing, a registered nurse (RN) already took the lead for pain management in each ward or department, and they were the most obvious choice of nurses to involve, as they had credibility in this area, and everyone would naturally look to them for leadership related to pain management (Golden 2006). However, this would not necessarily give representation to healthcare assistants (HCAs), whom Atwal and Jones (2007) have suggested are not always well recognised in discussions of multidisciplinary working. Alison was aware that the HCAs were often the people who did a great deal of the day-to-day assessment of pain, and who asked for patients to receive analgesia, or decided that this was not necessary. She therefore wanted to involve them in developing the protocol. There were six surgical wards in total, and theatres and the recovery area. If an RN and HCA were included from each area, it would become rather a large group. Alison and Charlotte therefore decided to involve the link nurses for pain from each area and a total of three HCAs. The HCAs were selected from the surgical wards as these were the areas where they would have most influence in pain management.

The pharmacist who would be involved was the senior pharmacist with overall responsibility for the surgical directorate, who would then cascade the information to their staff. They were the obvious choice as they would be the most constant and reliable presence, and whose agreement to a protocol would be seen as enduring. For similar reasons, the senior physiotherapist for the unit was chosen to represent physiotherapy, one of the senior ODPs was selected to represent his team and a medical technician volunteered to represent his discipline. These latter disciplines had one representative each as their day-to-day use of the protocol would be less than that of the nurses or medical staff.

The total number of people in the planning team stood at 20. Alison and Charlotte had wanted, if possible, to avoid a large group, as this can make interactions more problematic, with those who are most vocal likely to dominate (Atwal and Caldwell 2005). However, they had also tried to balance making the number manageable with taking into account who most needed to own and act on the change, and whether individuals or groups would feel intimidated or unable to contribute because of who the other group members were. Atwal and Caldwell (2005) suggest that perceived status can affect levels of participation in multidisciplinary meetings, and that medical staff may be the dominant force with other disciplines less likely to contribute. Although medical staff were vital, one of the reasons for reducing their number to four was that Alison felt that if they had the highest number of representatives, they would be more dominant and others might feel unable to put their point forward. The potential problem of HCAs being perceived as having lower status or experience in representing themselves at multidisciplinary meetings was still an issue, but Alison thought that as all the link nurses had to be involved, the lower number of HCAs was a necessary compromise.

Finally, patients and carers are increasingly seen as part of the multidisciplinary team (Royal College of Nursing and Royal College of Physicians 2006). Alison and Charlotte wondered about how they could meaningfully involve service users in the protocol development process. Patients who were currently on the wards were not thought to be suitable candidates because they were unlikely to be well enough to participate, so they decided to speak to the Patients' Advisory and Liaison Service (PALS) about the best way to involve ex-patients in developing the new protocol.

Mapping out which disciplines will be affected by a new way of working gives you an indication of who will need to be involved in planning change.

As well as thinking about who should be involved in change that affects the multidisciplinary team, and in what numbers, it is useful to consider whether all of the groups involved will hold equal weighting in planning and effecting each aspect of change. In an ideal world, a group will reach a consensus on each point about a new way of working, but this may not always be the case, and the leader of the change process may have to suggest, or guide, the group, as to whose opinion needs to count the most, either overall, or in specific instances. The reasons for such decisions will usually concern who is authorised to approve or disapprove the decision, whom the change in practice will have the greatest effect on, and whose ownership of it is essential. For example, Alison knew that unless the pharmacists agreed to what was being prescribed and medical staff were prepared to prescribe it, the rest of the pathway would be largely impossible to follow. As such, the views of medical staff and pharmacists had to hold the most weight in the prescribing element of the protocol, even if they did not for other aspects. The weighting of opinion may not always correlate with the number of people from each group who are involved: pharmacists held power of veto for any new prescription, but it was unnecessary for a large number of pharmacists to be involved because it would be enough that the senior pharmacist for the unit approved the protocol.

Who to Involve in Planning Multidisciplinary Change?
Who will need to work in the new way?
Who will be affected by the new way of working?

continued

Who will think they should be involved (and should they be)?
How many of each group need to be involved?
What will the number from each group mean for planning dynamics?
Does that give a manageable and representative total group size?

Some weighting also has to be given to the influence that people will have on the process of change as a whole, regardless of their professional affiliation. For example, if someone feels they should be involved at every level of the decision-making process, and are likely to be disgruntled and persuade others to work against the change if they are not, it may be expedient to seek more of their involvement than you actually need. Alison and Charlotte found that one of the surgeons had very strong views on the practicalities of the pain assessment documents. Although he was unlikely to be the person completing these, if his views on this were not seen to be listened to it was quite possible that he would oppose the whole protocol. Whilst Alison was not convinced that this was really within his remit, she was also aware that this particular surgeon had been asked to be on the group because, if he opposed the protocol, staff who worked with and around him would also be discouraged from using it. Thus, it was important to be seen to be taking his opinion on board, and giving it some weight, unless there was a compelling reason not to, even if it was not really merited on the grounds of his discipline's use of that part of the protocol. This was a part of considering who the key players and opinion leaders in each discipline were.

Planning successful multidisciplinary change includes making sure no one is missed, but also keeping the planning group to a manageable size.

Key Players and Opinion Leaders

For change that involves a multidisciplinary group to be effective, as well as the right disciplines being involved in planning the new way of working, those representing the disciplines have to be the right people. Alison and Charlotte considered, amongst other things, whether the individuals whom they were involving would: accurately represent the views of their discipline, do what they had agreed to do, promote the new protocol, and command the kind of relationship within their discipline and workplace, which would make their opinion count. In nursing, the link nurses for pain from each ward had an established role in relation to pain management, and would be the expected source of new information and the first route of enquiry for staff. Thus their formal position made them the obvious choice (Golden 2006). They would also be seen as credible sources of information and advice about pain management and would have the technical and theoretical skills and knowledge needed to work in the new way (Golden 2006). They might additionally know who would be likely to oppose or work with any initiative related to pain management, and be well placed to address this. Conversely, if one of them was not involved, it would undermine their role and might make them resist the new way of working, which would translate into their ward as a whole being unlikely to participate.

In other situations, there are not such obvious candidates to involve in planning multidisciplinary change, and thinking about who the opinion leaders in any discipline are, and asking others to make suggestions about whom to involve can be very useful (Iles and Cranfield 2004, Richens et al. 2004, Hall and Hord 2011: 221). When she was considering which HCAs to invite to join the team, Alison asked the link nurses if any HCAs on their wards were particularly interested in pain management, or particularly likely to oppose, challenge, or block the new way of working. As a result, she approached three suggested HCAs to join the group: two who were interested in pain management and would be likely to be influential in promoting this, and one who did not consider formal pain assessment to be important, and influenced other staff to follow her lead. This HCA was perhaps not the most obvious choice, but having her involved meant there was an opportunity for her to input into and own this way of working, which might mean that she would promote, rather than oppose, it. It might also give an opportunity for others on the development team to think about the arguments which anyone opposing the new way of working might bring, and enable the HCA concerned to learn more about her colleagues' views on pain assessment and management, and to perhaps see things differently.

An alternative approach to selecting people to participate in planning change is to seek volunteers, which was how the medical technician had been selected. This approach has pros and cons: volunteers are likely to have an interest in the subject, and being able to volunteer might mean that people who would not otherwise be thought of have a chance to participate. The downside of asking for volunteers is that although their interest may be valuable, those who do not have the confidence to put themselves forward are likely to be missed, and volunteers may not have the necessary skills, or be those who command respect or influence within their teams. However, asking for volunteers can be a useful way of engaging individuals, and keeping on board those who have an interest in the matter in question.

Although it is important to identify key players in each discipline, individuals often have influence across professional boundaries, and these influences, as well as discipline-specific issues, need to be taken into account in planning change. The HCA who had been invited to join the group mainly because she saw pain assessment as low priority was an opinion leader as defined by Hall and Hord (2011: 221) in that her views tended to affect how others thought and acted. She was likely, on a day-to-day basis, to influence whether junior doctors wrote prescriptions, and how nursing staff, especially junior nurses, assessed and managed pain. Hall and Hord (2011: 221) identify that opinion leaders may not be high profile or senior members of staff, and in this case, the HCA concerned was a key player across disciplines, despite being in a group, which might not be seen as high within the official hierarchy of healthcare staff. At the same time, she liked and respected the second anaesthetist who was on the protocol development group, and it was possible that his support for any new protocol would convince her to accept and promote it.

A key but also complex part of planning change that affects a number of different disciplines is having the right disciplines, the right people from that discipline, and also the right people in general terms, involved. Although the focus is often on the discipline- and profession-specific issues involved in multidisciplinary change management, each profession and discipline is made up of individuals, whose interactions and views may be at group, individual, or discipline-specific levels. A part of working to successfully effect change that involves this complex combination is to be very clear about, and stay focused on, the aim of the project.

Disciplines are made up of people: getting the right people from each discipline involved in change is as important as involving the right disciplines.

The Aim of Change

Whilst you are managing the complexity of multidisciplinary change, keeping a clear vision of your primary aim can help you to make focused decisions about which agendas you can take on board or absorb. The aim of Alison and Charlotte's work was to agree a new protocol for post-operative pain assessment and management, which would be used from theatre to discharge. The protocol itself was not an option, although what went into it, who contributed to it, how it was designed, rolled out, and implemented day to day, were open to negotiation. The planned meetings were intended to achieve this aim. Whilst group members were likely to wish to discuss other associated issues during meetings, having a clear aim would mean that conversations could be more easily redirected back to it. This might be particularly important in multidisciplinary meetings, as they had the potential to afford an opportunity for general resolution of issues between disciplines, or discussion of other projects, which was rarely available. Whilst goodwill was important, and a certain amount of flexibility in discussions might be needed, equally vital would be keeping a focus on the task in hand.

Summary

Managing change in healthcare very often involves developing a new way of working that requires the input of practitioners from across professions and disciplines. Planning and implementing change that involves a variety of disciplines draws on the same principles as all change management. However, it also requires consideration of why different disciplines need to be involved, which disciplines this should include, what their level of input should be, and which type of staff and which individuals from each group will most enhance the chance of successful change. This includes thinking about the interests, skills, attributes, and influence that people will have within their own disciplinary group and across disciplines. Finally, keeping focused on the aim of the proposed change is important, so that whilst appropriate alterations to the original plan can be made, the core aim remains the mainstay of any new way of working.

Key Points

Identifying which disciplines need to be involved in a proposed change is necessary.

Planning successful multidisciplinary change includes identifying key players in each discipline.

Disciplines are made up of people, and selecting the right people from each discipline to involve in planning change is vital.

Having clear aims for an innovation should enable you to work with the agendas and priorities of different disciplines, without losing the focus of the new way of working.

CASE STUDY

Soraya works on a unit that caters for young people with learning disabilities. The unit includes a residential area, day care facilities, an assessment and treatment area, and a small school. A number of the young people who access the unit have behaviour problems, and Soraya recently became interested in a new approach to behaviour management. She investigated the evidence to support this, and found that it could be an effective approach for many of the young people whom she works with. However, for it to be effective, everyone working with the children concerned would need to use it consistently. Because of this, Soraya considered how she could involve people from across all the relevant disciplines in exploring if, and how, the new approach could be implemented. In her initial thoughts, she considered the following points.

What Type of Team Was Involved?

The team concerned was a multidisciplinary team: they co-operated and communicated well with one another, and made joint plans for the input, which the young people needed, but each discipline had specific and separate functions, and there was relatively little blurring of professional boundaries.

The intention of the new behaviour management approach was not to change or challenge the existing division of roles, but for all the disciplines involved to use this approach when they worked with the young people for whom it might be beneficial.

Which Professions or Disciplines Should Be Involved?

Soraya thought about who would be the key manager of behaviour in each situation that a young person might be in, because these were the people who would need to be involved. From this she identified that:

RNs would need to be involved, because they planned and managed the day-to-day care that the young people needed, and led in providing their hands on care.

HCAs would need to be involved, as they provided a great deal of the day-to-day care that the young people needed.

Occupational therapists, speech and language therapists, and physiotherapists would need to be involved, as they often worked one to one with the young people, and would need to be able to instigate behaviour management during assessment or therapy sessions.

Social care staff often had input into the young people's day-to-day care, and took those who used the residential area on outings. They therefore needed to be involved.

Teaching staff would need to be involved, as they managed the young people's behaviour in the school setting.

Although the unit had a residential area, this was mainly used for short break care. The majority of young people spent most of their time with their own or foster families. Thus, for any new approach to behaviour management to achieve its potential, families, and in particular the young people's parents or foster parents, would need to be prepared to use, and therefore needed to be involved in discussions of, any new way of working.

Why Would These Disciplines' Involvement Be Useful?

The disciplines that Soraya had identified were all regularly involved in the direct care and supervision of the young people concerned. They would all be instrumental in making approaches to behaviour management consistent. If this was not achieved, any approach was less likely to work.

Involving all the disciplines that would be required to use any new approach to behaviour management at the discussion stage would mean that their views on the idea itself, its practicality, and any issues that it might present would be able to be discussed. This discussion would also enable staff from different disciplines, and the young people's parents and foster parents, to hear what the views of and issues for each other might be, so that the final decision, the reasons for this, and the challenges it might present were known by all concerned. A part of this discussion might include what training, skills, and expertise each group already had, and any additional input they might need.

Involving all the groups who would be most concerned in the new way of working in planning it might also enable potentially differing beliefs, values, priorities, and assumptions that existed about young people's behaviour to be identified, and discussed. This was likely to be important, as individual and group beliefs, priorities, and assumptions were likely to affect how they managed behaviour.

Involving representatives from across disciplines would enable the likely readiness for change amongst each group, other competing priorities and demands they were facing, and any recent changes that they had undergone, which might affect this initiative to be identified. It would also mean that people would be able to receive information from representatives of their own discipline, and that each discipline would have a change champion or champions.

Which Staff, and How Many from Each Group, Should Be Involved?

There was one occupational therapist, one physiotherapist, and one speech and language therapist designated to cover the unit, so they were the obvious choices to involve for their discipline. One teacher provided input at the school. She had support from a teaching assistant two days a week, but managed the classroom environment, and was therefore again the obvious choice. To organise the social care worker's involvement, Soraya decided to discuss the matter with two of the social care support staff who frequently worked with the young people on the unit, and ask their views about who to involve.

From the nursing staff, Soraya thought that two additional RNs and three HCAs might be a good number. One of the RNs on the unit worked mainly night shifts, and although involving her could be difficult because the planning meetings would happen in the day, Soraya considered that there would be advantages to her being on the group. It would be important to have consistent behaviour management day and night, and she knew that this nurse often felt excluded from discussions about developments on the unit, because of mainly working nights. This often led to her opposing new ideas and Soraya thought that inviting her to participate might help to bring her on board with this initiative. It would also mean that there was an opportunity to highlight issues that were specific to night shifts, which not all staff might know about. Another RN had been on the unit for a very long time, and was an opinion leader amongst staff and parents. Having her on board would be instrumental in the project's success or otherwise. These were the members of staff whom Soraya thought she would invite to represent the RNs.

One HCA on the unit was particularly interested in behaviour management, and always wanted to explore the best way to approach this, so he was a clear choice for Soraya to invite to participate. Another was undertaking an NVQ qualification and was studying a unit on change and innovation: Soraya thought being involved in this project might be useful for her NVQ work, and make any effort required to undertake a new way of working a part of an existing project. She also identified one HCA who informally acted as a liaison with parents, often spent a great deal of time with them, and who they always asked for. Although she also wanted parent representation, she felt that having this person on the group might make it easier for parents to express their views, and this HCA might also know about and be able to contribute further parental perspectives.

Parents were going to be a very important part of any change in practice related to behaviour management. The key question for Soraya was how many parents to include, and whom to include. The unit had a parent's link group, which had three parent representatives, and Soraya felt that the logical way forward would be to approach these parents and see if they wanted to participate, or knew of other parents who would like to. She thought that those who already acted as parent representatives might understand the representation role best, and might already have established communication channels with other parents. However, she also recognised that they might be over-committed, and that other people might want to become involved. At the same time, if she did not ask these three parents, they might feel that their roles as representatives were being undermined. She asked the HCA who she had noticed had an informal liaison role with parents her views, and discovered that one mother was already using this approach to behaviour management with her son. Soraya decided that she would be an important person to involve, as well as asking the three who were already parent representatives their views on who else to invite.

Should Equal Weighting Be Given to Everyone's Opinion?

Soraya's opinion was that those who would most often need to instigate any new approach to behaviour management should have the greatest influence. If those who were required to work, and take the lead day to day, in a new approach to behaviour management did not feel inclined to do so, it would fail. This meant that the views and final opinions of RNs, HCAs, the teacher, and parents or foster parents in particular would all be critical. The other groups would also be important, but did not have as much consistent day-to-day input with the young people.

Who Were the Key Players in Each Discipline?

Soraya considered the influence which each person she thought of involving would have within their own discipline, and across disciplines. The RN whom she wanted to invite to participate because of her influence amongst staff was influential across all staff groups, and also had some influence with parents. The HCA who had been selected because of her liaison with parents was likely to be a key influence with parents as well as some of her colleagues. The physiotherapist who usually covered the unit, whilst the only possible representative from her discipline, was known by staff and parents for seeing effective behaviour input as important, and insisting that the young people adhered to any behavioural regime they were using. Thus, her buy in to any new way of working related to behavioural issues was likely to enhance its acceptance across staff and parent groups. Despite not being based on the unit, and not having so much day-to-day contact with the young people like some other disciplines, she was an opinion leader in terms of behaviour management, and her view was likely to carry significant weight.

GUIDED WORK

This section revisits the learning outcomes covered in the chapter. You may want to complete it alone, or with colleagues.

1. Distinguish multidisciplinary, interdisciplinary, and transdisciplinary working.

- List the different disciplines in the team you work in, and the roles they fulfil.
- Does the way your team function most closely match a multidisciplinary, interdisciplinary, or transdiciplinary approach?

2. Identify whether more than one discipline needs to be involved in a given innovation.

Identify a change that you would like to implement.

- Decide which disciplines would need to be involved in planning this innovation.
- Why would these disciplines need to be involved?

3. Decide which individuals from different disciplines should take on key roles in change.

For the change that you identified above, consider:

- How many people from each discipline should be involved, and why.
- Whether equal weighting would be given to every discipline's opinion, or if there are some areas in which one discipline should lead.
- Which individuals should be involved from each discipline, and why.
- Who the key players and opinion leaders in each discipline are.
- Who these key players and opinion leaders might influence (within their own discipline and in other groups)?
- How you would gain their support.

4. Appreciate the potential complexity of managing individual and group agendas and concerns in planning and implementing change.

For the change you identified above:

- What would your main aim be?
- Are there any parts of the innovation that particular disciplines or individuals might object to?

- Could you modify these without losing sight of your aim?
- Are there any parts of your innovation that other might want to 'hijack' for their own aims?
- How far could you compromise to gain their co-operation without losing your focus?

Additional Resources

Inter-professional change management:
http://ipe.utoronto.ca/docs/IMPLC_Toolkit_Section_7.pdf

Mental health commission discussion paper on multidisciplinary working:
http://www.mhcirl.ie/documents/publications/Discussion%20Paper%20Multidisciplinary%20Team%20Working%20%20From%20Theory%20to%20Practice%202006.pdf

Report on multidisciplinary approaches to public health:
http://www.vha.org.au/uploads/multi-disciplinaryapproachesinphmay2005.pdf

8

Evaluating Change

Chapter Learning Outcomes

After studying this chapter, the reader will be able to:

- Determine the right time to evaluate various elements of change
- Understand a range of approaches to, and methods of, evaluating change
- Select an appropriate way to interpret the information gathered in evaluation activities
- Appreciate the ethical issues involved in the evaluation of change.

Summary

This chapter discusses processes and strategies that can be adopted in evaluating change, including evaluation of whether change has happened, its effect, and the reason for its success or otherwise; the timing of evaluation; approaches to evaluation; methods that may be used to conduct evaluation; selecting who to involve in collecting and analysing evaluative information; approaches to analysing information; and the ethics of evaluation. It concludes by identifying the need to see evaluation as the beginning of the next stage of practice development rather than an end point.

Claire works as a community nurse, and has a particular interest in people who have dementia. Carers often complain to her that they have very little choice about the timing of their short-break care. Because of this, and after discussions with carers and staff, Claire has piloted a system whereby carers are advised of how much short-break care they have been assessed as being entitled to, and can use an online system to make requests for their slots. The available short-break care slots are shown on a rota, and carers can see what other requests (which are anonymised) have been made, and then make their own requests. Claire has just carried out the six month post implementation evaluation.

Why Evaluate Change?

Evaluation of change is necessary, because, having instigated a new way of working, you need to know whether or not it is happening, and whether it has improved things, left them much the same as they were, or made them worse (Skinner 2004, Cork 2005, Welford 2006, Reid et al. 2007). For Claire, it was important to know whether the new way of booking short-break care was being used, whether it was useful for carers, and workable for staff.

Even if it seems as though it will be obvious whether or not you have achieved the aims of changing practice, and whether the new way of working is beneficial, having evidence of this is useful. If an evaluation of change shows positive outcomes, it can be used to justify the continued use of a new system, address criticisms, and seek ongoing support. If the evaluation shows that the new way of working is not beneficial, this evidence can enable you to abandon something that is not working, and explain in the future why the approach has not been taken. Carers had often asked Claire why they could not choose when they had short-break care, and one of her aims in piloting this system was to see whether, in reality, it was workable. If it was, then it might be a useful development, but if not, having evidence of this would enable her to explain to families that it had been tried, and why it could not be offered.

Conducting a formal evaluation should give you an objective and impartial insight into a new way of working. When your project appears to have been successful, a detailed evaluation can confirm this, and sometimes highlight areas where you could make things even better. In addition, evaluating the process as well as the outcome of change can show you what it was that made this change in practice work. Alternatively, if you think that an innovation has not gone well, you may find that things are not quite as bad as you think, and if things have not gone to plan, an evaluation may help you to identify why this is (Pryjmachuk 1996, Skinner 2004).

Although Claire had had her doubts about the new system, she now felt that, despite some initial problems, it was appreciated by carers, and less problematic for staff than had been anticipated. However, she wanted to check whether this really was the case, and thought that before suggesting that they offer the system more widely she would need evidence of whether it really did work, and was beneficial. She also wanted to glean a full picture of the pros and cons of the system, because some problems that could be absorbed on a small pilot might be less manageable for a wider population.

Evaluating change should give you evidence of whether an innovation is really workable, and if it has led to any improvements.

What Should Be Evaluated?

Ideally, an evaluation of a new way of working should include whether the change in practice has happened, the process by which this was achieved, and its effect (Reid et al. 2007). Sometimes things are thought to have changed, but have not really, and evaluating change without knowing whether the new way of working is really happening may mean that you evaluate the effect of nothing. The first part of evaluating an innovation should therefore be designed to tell you whether or not anything really has changed (Hall and Hord 2011: 63). Claire had to ascertain whether the new system was being used before exploring whether or not those involved found it helpful. If not, she might have found that carers were all very satisfied during the pilot phase, and implemented the new system across a wider population, only to discover that the system had actually never been used during the pilot phase, and it was only by chance that people had been getting short-break care slots that fitted their needs well.

Some changes are implemented, but do not improve things for anyone, and the evaluation of change should therefore be designed to tell you not only whether the intended change has taken place, but also whether or not it is having a positive effect. Claire wanted to ascertain whether the new way of working gave carers better choices, and whether they found this beneficial. However, she also wanted to know what staff thought of the new system of booking short-break care, because even if it had advantages for carers, it had to be workable for staff in order to be sustainable.

Finally, to be really useful, an evaluation has to be able to ask why: why something is happening or not, works or does not, or is beneficial or not (Blamey and MacKenzie 2007). This enables you to check on whether the idea behind an innovation, the process of change, or factors extraneous to the change itself, might have affected its implementation, benefits, or perceived value. Claire's early evaluation when she rolled out the new system for booking short-break care showed that the person doing the rota found the new approach very labour intensive. On exploring this further, Claire discovered that the system had some compatibility issues with the computer system that this person was using, which could easily be resolved. If she had not asked 'why' she would have concluded that the system was cumbersome and unworkable. By asking why, she was able to find a solution that could easily be effected.

A good evaluation should ask whether or not change has been implemented, what effect it has had, and why.

What to Evaluate

1. Has change been implemented or not?
   If not: why not?
   If yes: what facilitated this?
2. What has happened because of the new way of working?
   Include positive and negative outcomes.
   Think about unexpected outcomes.
3. Why have there been these outcomes?

Having clear aims and objectives for an innovation assists in designing the evaluation, because it means that you know what you need to evaluate. Claire's aim had been to find out if there is any benefit in carers making their requests for short breaks via an online system, which shows what is available, and what other requests have been made.

Her objectives had been

- to see if this approach to booking short-break care is practically possible;
- to see if this approach to booking short-break care is beneficial for carers;
- to see if this approach to booking short-break care is workable for staff.

This meant that, at the end of the project, she needed to evaluate whether using such a system was practical, whether carers found it beneficial, and whether staff found it workable. However, within each of these objectives, she also needed to define the terms used.

Claire decided that, for her project, 'practical' meant whether the system was sufficiently straightforward that people were prepared to use it, and that the requisite equipment was available to those who needed it. To evaluate this, she needed to see if people used the system or not, and why. The why for this point was important, for example, to distinguish whether any families who were not using the system did not want to make requests, did not know about the system, had forgotten about it, or did not find it user friendly enough.

For her second objective, of ascertaining whether this system was bene-ficial for carers, Claire had to define what she deemed to be beneficial. She defined this as including whether the carers felt that they had more choice in when care was provided, had a better awareness of why they could not always be offered the care slots that they would like, and whether they were able to plan their time and other commitments better. She also wanted to know if they liked having this choice, and if there were any disadvantages to it.

In terms of whether the new system was workable for staff, Claire felt that she had two main issues to explore. Firstly, whether the person who did the rota found the system workable. This was a very important point as a major issue was likely to be whether the requests from families made the job of devising the staff rota more or less problematic. However, as well as the perspectives of the person writing the rota, Claire wanted to get the views of the staff that had to work the rotas produced. The main things she thought she needed to explore with staff were whether the new system affected their rotas, the continuity of their care provision, and whether they saw any changes as positive or negative. How she explored these aspects of the new system is discussed in the section on methodology and methods.

Evaluation should be designed to assess whether or not your intended aims and objectives have been achieved.

As well as checking whether or not change has happened, evaluating whether it is beneficial, and why, the timing of evaluation influences how accurate a picture of the effect and effectiveness of the new way of working it provides.

When to Evaluate

If the change you are implementing has several stages, you should aim to carry out some form of evaluation at every stage: there is no point in mov-ing to stage two of your plan if you are not sure if stage one has happened, particularly if stage two depends on stage one having been completed suc-cessfully. This will also help you to evaluate the process of change, because you will be able to identify any stages where problems were encountered, delays experienced, resources limited, or where key events went particularly well. The first part of Claire's plan was to discuss the idea of the new method of booking short-break care with carers and staff to see if they would consider it. If all the carers had stated that, despite the advantages, the effort required to use this system would be too much on top of their other responsibilities, there would have been no benefit in pursuing the idea. Claire had therefore needed to check whether this consultation stage was complete, and what the findings from it were, before she moved on to the next stage of planning the processes involved. The evaluation at this stage was a list of all the carers she proposed for the pilot, and staff who would be involved, with a tick against those whom she had spoken to and a note stating whether the carers and staff were interested in being a part of the pilot or not.

It was also useful at this stage for Claire to investigate some whys. Some staff were not very keen on the idea because they felt that it would mean that carers could request care at any time, and that their own working hours would change or have to be more flexible. This indicated to Claire that she needed to emphasise to all parties that the hours that were available, and already being worked, would be offered out for carers to make their requests from. It also clarified to her that whilst some staff might seem opposed to the new system, the concept of carers making choices was not necessarily problematic, but how it was implemented would be important. In the longer term, Claire thought that the system might be able to be used to offer staff as well as careers more flexibility, but this was a step too far at this point in time.

Although evaluating every stage of a change in practice is important, the final stage is often where the most comprehensive evaluation needs to be: this is where you have introduced the change in practice in its entirety and want to know if it works. The timing of the final evaluation of change usu-ally requires more thought than the preceding stages. The interim stages are usually progressive, and the evaluation happens logically as each stage ends, before proceeding to the next. Although there may be delays at any stage of planning and implementing change, which create reciprocal delays in the timing of the evaluation, the schedule is essentially set. However, when you consider when to carry out the final evaluation of a new way of working, you need time for the change in practice to have happened, to have shown an effect, and to have overcome any natural teething problems that might conceal its real worth.

Claire had to wait long enough for the new way of working to affect provision of short-break care, as well as requests, before she could evalu-ate its worth. She could have evaluated within three months whether the practicalities of the rota in terms of people having access to the system, mak-ing requests, and a rota being issued, which took these into account had been achieved. However, whether or not people found this useful and workable would be better assessed when carers had had a reasonable exposure to the process and product of the new way of booking short-break care, and staff had become a little more accustomed to it. Claire also wanted to wait long enough for any initial problems to have been addressed. She felt that by evaluating at six months, the staff and families concerned would effectively have at least three months experience of using the whole system.

Planning that enables evaluation at the end point of an innovation is important, so that you know whether to continue to use it or not. However, it is usually a good idea not to rely entirely on the time just after new practice has been introduced to evaluate whether it is happening and whether it works well. An initiative may initially work well, especially if you have had the time and resources to invest in encouraging people to participate and checking that they are doing so. As time goes by, people's enthusiasm may lessen, other priorities come along, what was working well starts to stumble, and slowly everyone reverts to the old way of doing things (Balasubramanian et al. 2010). To avoid this, or to pick up on whether it is happening, it may be useful to plan short-term, medium-term, and ongoing evaluations. If the evaluation at six months showed that the system was working well enough to merit continuation, Claire planned to evaluate the pilot again after a year. If it was still working well, she intended to expand it to a larger group, and re-evaluate after 18 months and then two years. As Chapter 10 will discuss, this can help to sustain change by maintaining your own and other people's interest in the project, and can also help you to identify if practice has really changed, and whether the new way of working is sustainable.

Evaluate

At the end of every stage of an innovation
Early enough to facilitate feedback and sustain interest
When there will have been time for the effects of change to be evident
Beyond the honeymoon period

Evaluation of change should not be a one-off event.

How to Evaluate Change: Evaluation Design and Methods

The right way to evaluate change depends on what you are evaluating. To make this decision, it is useful to look at the aim(s) or objective(s) that you are evaluating, the nature of these, whether you are assessing if change has happened, or its effect, and from this decide what sort of information you need (Comfort 2010). If you are evaluating an aim that would be best assessed using numerical measurement, then your evaluation should use methods of gathering information that will achieve this. These methods may draw on similar principles to those of quantitative research, because they aim to quantify facts (McGrath and Johnson 2003, Lee 2006). If, on the other hand, what you need to know is more concerned with personal experiences, views, attitudes, or values then you probably need to use methods that draw on qualitative research approaches (Kearney 2005, Reid et al. 2007). Many evaluations will use a combination of approaches, because different aspects of new practice will need to be evaluated.

To evaluate her first objective, Claire sought to identify whether or not the change in practice that she was proposing was practical. A part of this was to find out whether or not the new booking system was being used. To achieve this she measured, from the electronic records, how many carers who were in the pilot scheme were using the new system. She also wanted to know how many of the requests made were met, and again, she evaluated this numerically, comparing the requests made with the published rotas.

As well as seeing whether people used the system or not, Claire wanted to know carers' and staff views on its practicality, and to explore in some depth why people did or did not use it. This would be best achieved by discussing with those concerned their experience of using the system, what worked for them and what did not. For this part of evaluating her first objective, Claire used the principles of qualitative enquiry, with semi-structured interviews as her evaluation method.

Claire's initial quantitative evaluation told her whether the change in practice appeared to have happened, and some of the information from it helped her to design the schedule for her discussions with families and staff. Her overall approach therefore drew on the principles of mixed methods research, using a sequential design, in which the first, quantitative, stage of data collection informed the second, qualitative, aspect (Creswell 2003, Tashakkori and Teddlie 2003, Mertens 2005, Curry et al. 2009). A mixed methods approach is often useful in evaluation, because it allows different aspects of a situation to be explored, and reasons for the success or otherwise of innovations to be shown (Garbarino and Holland 2009).

The approach to evaluation that you use should be determined by the type of information you need.

Approaches to Evaluation: Checklist

For every stage of an innovation ask yourself:

What do you need to evaluate?
Will it be best assessed using numbers, in-depth descriptions or accounts, or a
    combination of these?

Approaches to Evaluation: Checklist *continued*

What is the best way to get the information you need (for example, observing, talking to people, looking at records or charts, and distributing a questionnaire)?

Will the approach you have chosen tell you not only what happened, but also why?

As well as thinking about what type of information you want, you have to decide how you will get that information, and decisions about this should be guided by what type of information you are looking for. There are no right or wrong evaluation methods: it depends on what you are evaluating. You might use questionnaires, observation, analysis of documents, interviews (with individuals or groups), pre- and post-tests, and many more. Whichever tool or tools you use need to be designed to assess, measure, or investigate exactly what you want to know about (Reid et al. 2007). When Claire was evaluating her first objective, whether the new system for booking short-break care was practical, she wanted to see who had and had not made requests for short-break care, and if these have been met. To do this, she used the records of requesting and rotas. As well as deciding that she wanted to measure whether or not people used the system, Claire had to decide whether she wanted to measure how many families used it, or how many times they used it. She also had to decide if all that she wanted to measure was overall numbers or whether she wanted to break this down further, for example, to distinguish between those using the system for weekend care and those using it for slots of a few hours. However, although your evaluation strategy should be designed to accommodate every point that might require evaluation or comparison, there is also benefit in not making the potentially simple complex unless you have to. Claire carried out an overall check to see if there were any short-break sessions for which requests had not been made before deciding whether or not to measure if there were differences in the type of short-break care requested. If 100% of short-break care sessions were requested via the new system, then wondering who was and was not using the system would be pointless. It can be worth getting the overall picture before worrying too much about the minutiae, because you may not need to.

To find what staff and carers thought of the new system Claire decided to use semi-structured interviews, because she thought that this would enable her to explore in some depth why they did or did not use the new system, and what they thought of it. She considered using questionnaires, but decided that as the number of people involved in the pilot was fairly small, using a face-to-face approach was achievable. She was not sure that people would include the depth of information that she hoped to gain in responses to a questionnaire, or that they would complete the questionnaires, but thought that they probably would agree to discuss their experiences with her. She used semi-structured, rather than structured, interviews, so that she would be able to follow up leads and ideas that developed during conversations or as the evaluation progressed. She did not want to use unstructured interviews, because she wanted to keep her discussions focused on the new system for booking short-break care, not other aspects of support (Burck 2005, Whiting 2008). Claire also considered using group interviews, but because of the care needs of clients and the rotas staff worked, this was likely to be impractical. Thus, her decision about method was based in part on ideals and in part on what was practical and achievable.

It is useful to think about whether your evaluation needs to capture any differences between rhetoric, intentions, beliefs, and what actually happens in practice (Haveri 2008). Claire thought it possible that carers would feel obliged to say they used the system, because, having complained about the previous system, they felt that they should. By using an evaluation strategy that included talking to staff and carers, and checking the records on the computer systems, she could determine whether people actually did use the system, as well as whether they said that they did.

There are no right or wrong evaluation tools, but there are tools that are right or wrong for a particular job.

You also have to decide on the sample of the people or events that will be involved in an evaluation of new practice. Claire had conducted a small pilot study, and as such felt that she could include everyone who had been involved in the evaluation. However, if the project had been larger, she might only have been able to sample the rotas, requests, and views of a selection of those involved, and would have had to decide how to choose which to select. She might have decided to use a form of probability sampling, in which each person who had been involved had an equal chance of being included in the sample that were chosen for the evaluation. However, although probability sampling, which usually involves randomisation, is often seen as the best approach in quantitative research, it is not usually used in qualitative enquiry, where the intention is to explore in some depth the particular perspectives of individuals.

Qualitative approaches to enquiry often use non-probability sampling, where not everyone has an equal chance of being selected and in which randomisation is not used. This might be achieved using purposive sampling, where participants are chosen deliberately, sometimes because they had a particular experience or are likely to have a particular way of viewing a situation (McGrath and Johnson 2003, Astin 2009). For the qualitative part of her evaluation, where Claire wanted to know what encouraged or stopped people from using the new system, it might have been useful for her to target a sample that included some carers who had used the system regularly, some who had used it occasionally, some who had never used it, and one or two who had experienced particular problems, to enable her to explore all these views.

Whilst purposive sampling can be useful, it means that people who have a particular experience, or view, may not get the chance to share it because they are not chosen. Claire might also have chosen another type of non-probability sample, such as a volunteer sample. If she had asked for volunteers, she would probably have got those who liked the system and wanted to say so, and those who wanted to complain, but few people whose opinions were 'middle of the road'. Each of these, and other approaches to selecting a sample for evaluation, has benefits and problems, which have to be weighed up. Your job as the person designing the evaluation is to choose the best sample for the job: the one that will get the most accurate information about what you want to evaluate, whilst also being achievable.

Often you also have to decide between the ideal and the manageable: purposive sampling may sometimes be the ideal, but be time consuming in terms of selecting, contacting, and arranging to visit the chosen selection of participants, so if time and resources are limited, a volunteer sample may be the only available option. When you analyse your evaluation information, the decisions you made about sampling will influence the way you interpret your findings, and the confidence with which you make any recommendations. If Claire had used a volunteer sample, in which it transpired that only those who used the new system regularly volunteered, she would have needed to include in her findings that the views on those who used the system intermittently or not at all were not known, rather than suggesting that her findings represented views from across the board.

Sometimes a change in practice brings outcomes that were not expected, and which have therefore not been catered for in the planned evaluation strategy (Reed and Turner 2005). Because you will not know what the evaluation will show, you need to be flexible about altering your approach to evaluation as you go, and to design strategies that can cater for things that you might not have considered. For example, one carer told Claire that using the new system had increased her confidence in using her computer. This was an unexpected positive outcome of the innovation, which was worth noting. Because Claire had used semi-structured interviews to explore the views of carers and staff, this type of issue could be identified and discussed, in a way that a highly structured interview schedule would probably not have allowed for (Burck 2005, Whiting 2008).

Whilst a planned evaluation strategy is important, if you are evaluating real-world events, in your own workplace, you are likely to have the option of unplanned evaluation opportunities. These are often very valuable and the fact that they are not included in your planned strategy does not mean that you should ignore them (Skinner 2004, Reid and Turner 2005). Claire had heard 'on the grapevine' that some of her colleagues were concerned that one family was trying to coerce others to meet their requirements before submitting their requests. This was something, which families might have found difficult to tell her, but she was able to use the information to cross-check who had requested what and when, and to provide some direction for planning her discussions, without making assumptions. During her interviews with families, it transpired that what had been perceived as coercion by staff had been seen by some families as a useful pre-requesting discussion to simplify the formal requesting process.

When you are evaluating new practice, you will nearly always have to think about distinguishing what happens because of a change in practice from things that happen at about the same time but are not actually anything to do with the new way of working. This might include staffing levels, organisational change outside your project, competing priorities, and a whole host of other things (Blamey and Makenzie 2007). This makes the why questions very important: Claire found that one family appeared to have stopped using the system, but when she explored the reason for this, she discovered that they had been experiencing problems with their Internet connection, but were still very keen to use the system once they were back online.

> *Evaluation should be designed to capture unexpected events, and to distinguish what happens because of innovation, and things that happen at the same time, but are not related to it.*

Who Should Evaluate

The person or people gathering the information that will be used to evaluate a new way of working can affect the quality of the evaluation (Skinner 2004). Your decisions about who will fulfil this role are therefore important. The ideal might be for you to gather all the information yourself. However, if this is not a realistic task for one person, you will have to enlist assistance. If more than one person is collecting the information, then you need to be sure that everyone is evaluating as close as possible to the same thing in the same way. This may be relatively easy if you are simply recording whether or not documents are used, or systems accessed, but it may sometimes be necessary to be very clear about what is being evaluated, and how the evaluation is to be conducted. Claire decided that she would be able to gather all the information for the evaluation of her project. If she had used a second person, they would have had to agree on what information they should gather about the requests that were made and the rotas, how the interviews would be conducted, what they aimed to discuss, and what the acceptable level of flexibility in the semi-structured schedule was.

Another issue to consider is whether the person collecting the information will affect what people say or do (Comfort 2010). Claire knew that people might not tell her what they really thought about the new system: they might not want to hurt her feelings, feel unable to criticise her project to her face, and if they were deliberately trying to sabotage the project it was unlikely that they would tell her this. She also worked with the families concerned, and was aware that, because the system had been developed as a result of requests for greater choice, they might feel obliged to give positive evaluations. They might also fear repercussions from criticising the system that she had set up. In addition, Claire was aware that she might find it difficult to ask people in a completely unbiased manner what they thought of the project, or why they were not using the new approach. She considered whether to get someone else to carry out the collection of information for the evaluation, particularly the interviews. The converse of this was that Claire was not convinced that another person would really know enough about the project to hold the evaluation conversations, or give completing it as high a priority as she did. Overall, she decided that she should collect the evaluative information, but was aware in planning and carrying out the evaluation activities that she would have to be careful to note any possible challenges created by her role and involvement in the process.

Although collecting information to evaluate your own project can create challenges, so can using other people to do this. If a manager is collecting the information, people may fear that it is being gathered to monitor their performance, rather than to evaluate the new way of doing things. In addition to the position and role of the person collecting the information, it is advisable to think about their skills and attributes. Depending on what type of information you need to collect, you may decide to look for someone who is skilled at using databases, or someone who is easy to talk to but also listens well and gains people's confidence quickly. Practically, you also need someone who has enough time for, and commitment to, the project to do the necessary work (Comfort 2010).

What Might Affect the Accuracy of an Evaluation?

The person collecting the information
When the information was collected
The way the information was collected
How questions were asked
The way the information was analysed
How the information was interpreted

Accuracy of Information

When you design an evaluation strategy, you need to think about things that might make the apparent findings inaccurate (Eccles et al. 2003). This may happen because of design flaws in the methods you use to evaluate, or in the process itself, for example, in the way that questions are asked. It may be difficult for you to be unbiased about your project, because you are likely to want it to work. If you have been allowed time and resources to make a change in practice there may be pressure on you to show that it has worked, is being done, or has created improvement of some kind (Comfort 2010). Whilst this may not mean that you would deliberately be dishonest in your evaluation, it does create pressure to show that things are working reasonably well. However, you have to be sure that you are setting up an evaluation that is designed to accurately assess how things are working, not to prove success.

Claire tried to word her evaluation questions very neutrally, and listened to all her recordings of interview conversations to see whether or not she had appeared to encourage staff or families to give positive responses, or whether anything in the tone of their response indicated that they felt obliged to give a positive evaluation. She also kept a record throughout the project of anything that might be a useful contribution to the evaluation, or might influence how she interpreted the information gathered (Roberts and Priest 2006). For example, she was aware that she viewed one member of staff as particularly difficult, and likely to oppose change, and wanted to be careful that she did not dismiss this person's views simply as a negative approach to change in general. After she analysed the information that she had gathered, she checked with the staff and families concerned whether she had interpreted what they said accurately. This is generally considered to be a good way of checking the accuracy of information gathered in qualitative research (Russell and Gregory 2003, Koch 2006, Roberts and Priest 2006). It can, however, bring with it a difficulty if your interpretation and that of participants is significantly at odds. To address this, it is useful to decide in advance what level of interpretation you will invite participants to comment on, for example, whether you are checking that the transcript of a discussion accurately reflects what they said and felt, or whether you are inviting them to comment on your interpretation of this information.

If other people are involved in carrying out an evaluation of change, you have to consider their possible biases as well as your own. Chapter 7 highlighted the possibility of inviting people who do not really support a change in practice to join a project team in order to increase their enthusiasm. It can be useful to remember this when you are designing the evaluation, and to perhaps ensure that they are not solely responsible for evaluating a part of the project that they never really supported in the first place. Equally, if someone has been very enthusiastic about a new way of working, and personally likes it, it may be worth considering their positive biases and building in mechanisms to guard against these influencing the evaluation. The aim of evaluation is to gain an accurate interpretation of what has happened, and to avoid anything in the methods and practicalities of the evaluative process detracting from this.

The information you gather to evaluate the effect of an innovation needs to provide an accurate reflection of what has happened, and why, so that future practice is directed on a sound basis.

Analysing Information

Gathering information has to be followed by deciding what this information means: how you do this depends on what type of information you collect (Glenaffric Ltd 2007).

If you have gathered numerical data, it needs to be dealt with using numerical means. Sometimes how you will interpret the information that you have gathered is very straightforward: when Claire evaluated the electronic rota requests, she only needed to check how many families used this system, and for how many of their total short-break care episodes. Although Claire was using a quantitative approach, as with many evaluations that involve just one team, ward, or unit, she did not need to, and could not realistically, get into any depth of statistical analysis. Instead, she used descriptive statistics in the form of raw scores and percentages (Windish and Diener-West 2006). This is usually completely acceptable, because you are not likely to have a large enough sample to do more, and because you only want to see if the change in practice works in the environment you want to use it in, not to use a test that will tell you how generalisable the findings are. If you are carrying out a larger scale evaluation or an evaluation from which you intend to claim wide generalisations, then you need to think about using inferential statistics. However, you only need to do this if the scale or intention of your evaluation merits it. Measurements should be valid, and accurate, suitable for the issue in question, but not unnecessarily complex (Harvey and Wensing 2003). In Claire's case, using descriptive statistics was perfectly acceptable.

As well as deciding how to numerically analyse information, you have to decide what level of achievement is acceptable for you to continue with the innovation. Claire had to have some idea of how high or low an acceptable level of people using the new system was. If she found that 100% of families were using this approach, there would be no problem, but unless things were that good, she needed to decide what level would make it seem worth carrying on without much further intervention, what level would mean that more input was needed, and what level meant a major rethink.

If your data is qualitative, then the analysis needs to match this, for example, by looking at the information that you have and coding and categorizing it or arranging it into themes (Burla et al. 2008, Balls 2009, Campos and Turato 2009). If you are collecting more than one type of information, you need to consider how it will all link together. Claire had to decide how she would link scores related to whether the new system was used or not with the codes developed from the qualitative analysis. She decided that the information she gathered using different methods would inform one another, in terms of the quantifiable evidence giving her ideas for her interview schedule, and the two types of information giving a more complete picture than using one alone would. The quantitative information would give an overall view of how the system was used, with the quantitative part providing more in-depth analysis of particular issues and why people did or felt as they did.

Ethics and Evaluation

The ethical obligation that healthcare staff have to do good and to do no harm, some might argue, means that introducing new practice without investigating its outcomes is unethical, as you do not know the effect that it has on individual patients, groups of patients, and whether it is a valid continued use of resources (Hughes 2008). When you evaluate new practice, you have an ethical obligation to obtain and present as accurate as possible a picture of events, so that the recommendations that you make for the ongoing use of an innovation are a true reflection of its benefits and the challenges involved.

Although evaluation should comply with ethical principles, an evaluation of an innovation in practice will not usually require approval by an ethics committee, as it involves an intervention that has been introduced primarily to improve care provision, and of which evaluation is the natural conclusion, rather than an activity for its own end (National Patient Safety Agency and Research Ethics Service 2009). It is more likely that a change in practice as a whole, including the evaluation strategy, will require approval through local governance processes, before being implemented. This was the route Claire had pursued in her innovation in provision of short-break care.

The way in which evaluation of change is conducted should follow the principles of healthcare ethics in terms of respecting autonomy, doing good, doing no harm, and seeking justice (Beauchamp and Childress 2001). The principle of respect for autonomy may be particularly applicable in terms of the choice that individuals or groups have over participating in evaluation, and whether they give informed consent for this (Coughlan et al. 2007). Claire had gained consent from all the families who were participating in the pilot to her checking the requests they made, and to taking part in interviews. However, staff rotas were also looked at in the evaluation, and the staff whose names appeared on the rotas and the person who devised the rota had to be advised of this. Claire's colleagues were also invited to participate in interviews, and had to be given enough information to provide informed consent to do so, or to decline to participate. Claire needed to consider issues surrounding coercion to participate, fear of reprisals for non-participation or for what was said, confidentiality of information and how this information was stored, shared and used. Although she only wanted to know about rotas and people's views in order to evaluate the innovation in question, staff participants might fear that their views would be identifiable by managers and used as evidence in other contexts. Similarly, there was the potential for carers to feel that the support they received might be affected by their participation and what they said. Claire sought to reduce these concerns by explaining that the evaluation was only being conducted to see if the system worked, because if it did not it would not be beneficial to continue, and that whilst she had managed the project, it was not in her interests to think it worked or helped people if it did not. She was not able to promise participants anonymity, as she was conducting face to face interviews, and their actual names appeared on the rotas, but she was able to say that the information she gathered would be anonymised, and confidentiality maintained over individual identities and contributions. However, she also advised participants that although she would not divulge anyone's identity in her evaluation report, as the sample was small, and local, it was possible that anyone reading the report might recognise individuals.

In terms of benefit and harm, Claire felt that the concerns that staff or families had about participating in the evaluation were the main potential harm, and sought to minimise these as described above. The fate of the innovation largely rested on the findings from the evaluation, and whether the new system was adopted or not could be beneficial or harmful to staff and families. Thus, the evaluation needed to be a true and accurate representation of the effects of the new system, so that if it was beneficial it would be developed and used, and if not, not.

Meeting the ethical requirement for justice includes whether everyone has an equal chance to contribute to or be represented in evaluation activities. Claire invited all those who had been involved in the new way of working to participate in the evaluation, so that all views would be equally heard, and influence ongoing decision-making about the new system being more widely used. If not everyone had been involved in the evaluation, her decisions about sampling would have needed to include whether the ethical principle of justice was addressed.

When you are planning the process of evaluating change you should consider the benefit, potential harm, and justice of the steps you are taking, and whether or not it respects people's autonomy.

Summary

Evaluation of change should be designed to show whether an innovation in practice has been implemented, the effect that this has had, why it has had this effect, and provide some indication of what should be done next. Evaluation, whatever its outcome, should not signal the end of change, but be seen as a stage in ongoing service or practice development. If the evaluation shows that everything has gone well, and things are better than they were, then your next task is to think about how to keep things improved and improving. If it shows that things have not gone as well as you hoped then identifying why may give you some suggestions of what to do next, to either try to achieve the desired change in another way, or abandon it. If you do decide to abandon the new way of working, there may still be aspects of the change in practice that you attempted, which can be usefully adapted, or there may be unexpected beneficial outcomes, which can be developed instead of the original innovation. A change that has not worked out as planned does not necessarily mean that nothing has been gained, or nothing further needs to be done.

Key Points

Evaluation of change should include whether change has happened, its effect, and the reason for its success or otherwise.

The timing of evaluation is important in presenting an accurate picture of the effect of change.

The approach and methods used for evaluation should be guided by what is being evaluated.

Evaluation processes should produce findings that accurately reflect what happened because of an innovation.

Evaluation of an innovation should be seen as the beginning of the next stage of practice development.

CASE STUDY

Tamsin and Dave are public health practitioners, and recently developed a health promotion initiative to encourage teenagers to choose not to smoke. Their initiative involved facilitating workshops in schools with pupils in year 11, to encourage discussion about smoking, why people might want to start smoking, its perceived advantages, and its adverse effects.

The aim of the initiative was to increase young people's awareness of the adverse effects of smoking.

The objectives were

1. to run a weekly workshop on smoking awareness with pupils in year 11 over one half term;
2. to provide pupils with accurate information about the effects of smoking;
3. to enable pupils to challenge their own views about smoking;
4. to foster in pupils the skills to enable them to decline to participate in smoking.

If the workshops proved to be successful, the intention was to introduce them in more schools. However, because it was a new approach, Dave and Tamsin began with a pilot in two schools. They then formally evaluated this in order to ascertain if the initiative should be continued. Their evaluation included:

Had the Change Been Implemented?

To be able to evaluate the effectiveness of their initiative, Dave and Tamsin first needed to determine whether the workshops had happened. This mainly concerned objectives 1 and 2. To ascertain this they numerically evaluated how many sessions ran at each school, how many were missed, and how many pupils attended. If sessions had been cancelled, or missed by pupils, they wanted to find out why this was.

What Was the Effect of the Innovation?

When they designed their project, Dave and Tamsin considered what they could realistically hope to achieve. The ultimate outcomes of interest were those included in objectives 2, 3, and 4, regarding whether or not pupils had an accurate understanding of the possible effects of smoking, had been able to challenge their views on smoking, or choose to refrain from smoking as a result of the workshops.

To evaluate these objectives, Dave and Tamsin carried out a brainstorming and discussion session during the first workshop, focused on the pupils' knowledge of, views about, and what influenced their participation in smoking. This was followed by a similar discussion session during the last workshop, with the contributions made in each session compared. However, Dave and Tamsin were aware that pupils might simply report what they perceived to be the right answers, which might not reflect their real thoughts, or might not be sustained after the weekly input had finished. To try to overcome this, and to assess the longevity of any apparent positive outcomes, they planned to repeat this discussion session six months after the workshops, to see if any positive developments appeared to be sustained.

There were no reliable existing statistics of how many children in year 11 smoked, so it would be impossible to do a pre- and post-intervention comparison to see if the workshops had any direct effect on the number of young people who chose to smoke. As the sessions were intended to have an ongoing effect, it would also be necessary to compare their effectiveness in later years, as well as immediately, and the number of variables involved, as well as the timescale, made such a comparison almost impossible, certainly in the short term. Dave and Tamsin's evaluation was therefore focused on aspects of the workshops that they felt could be achieved and evaluated within a reasonable time frame.

Did the Process of Change Contribute to Its Success or Failure?

Dave and Tamsin wanted to evaluate the process as well as outcomes of their initiative, to give them some ideas about the reasons for any apparent successes or failures. They had used an action plan that gave a step-by-step description of what had to be done in order to achieve their aims, for example, when and with whom they had consulted, who they had sought permissions from, when and how they had secured rooms, and when and how parents and pupils had been made aware of the project. By looking back on how and when these milestones were achieved, the responses they had encountered, and any additional information they had recorded about the process of setting up the workshops, they were able to pinpoint any aspects of how the initiative was managed or evolved, which might have contributed to the level of success that was achieved.

When Was a Good Time for the Evaluation Take Place?

Although the formal evaluation of the initiative was made after the final workshop, Tamsin and Dave evaluated the milestones detailed in the action plan as they went, and monitored whether sessions took place, and the reasons for any cancellations, as the project progressed.

The final evaluation of the effect of the programme on pupil's knowledge, and apparent beliefs, values and skills was carried out at the final workshop. A follow-up evaluation was planned for six months later, to see if any positive effects had been sustained.

What Approaches Were Used in the Evaluation?

Dave and Tamsin had two main approaches to evaluation: one quantitative and one qualitative. The quantitative element measured how many sessions ran, and how many pupils attended. The second part of the evaluation was qualitative. This was comprised of two elements. The first was the brainstorming and discussion sessions with pupils at the last workshop, and six months after the last workshop. The intention of this part of the evaluation was to gather information regarding pupils' beliefs, values, attitudes, and knowledge, which would best be assessed using qualitative methodology. The second part of the qualitative aspect of evaluation was examination of diaries that Dave and Tamsin kept.

What Evaluation Methods Were Used?

The quantitative aspect of the evaluation was conducted using a standardised log of session times and attendance.

The qualitative aspect of evaluation used a semi-structured group discussion with pupils. Using a group discussion carried a risk that dominant members of the group would lead the interaction, and influence others. However, this was balanced against the group situation being how smoking decisions might in be reached, and thus possibly more closely represented the real world of decision-making than one to one discussions with pupils might. It might also enable pupils to prompt one other to recall their thoughts or feelings, and provide a richer discussion. As the ethos of the workshops had been working together, and discussing and sharing views, it was anticipated that pupils would be prepared for this. The ground rules of participation in the workshops had been established on the first day and these would also apply to the evaluation sessions. One to one discussions to explore pupils' knowledge and views after the workshops were considered, but it was thought that this approach was more likely to be intimidating, and to produce a socially desirable rather than true response, than the group situation would.

Throughout the development of the project, and the process of setting up and conducting the workshops, Dave and Tamsin kept diaries that included observations of processes and events that were or could be important in the project. These diaries were examined as a part of the qualitative aspect of the evaluation.

Were Any Unexpected Evaluation Opportunities Utilised?

Some unplanned evaluation opportunities and information were available to Dave and Tamsin, which gave them important information on the success or otherwise of the workshops. This included comments that were overheard between pupils at or after workshops, or comments made by staff. These observations or events were noted in the diaries that Dave and Tamsin used, so that the information was not lost.

How Was the Information that Was Gathered Analysed?

Quantitative information was analysed using raw scores, as the numbers involved meant that anything more ambitious would be unrealistic. The qualitative information was analysed using thematic analysis. The two types of evaluative data supported one another in providing a clearer overall picture of the practicality, effectiveness and sustainability of the workshops than one approach would. Some links between the two sets of information could also be made, for example, some of the diary entries or statements made in the discussions gave insight into why pupils had or had not attended, or sessions been cancelled.

Who Carried out the Evaluation?

Dave and Tamsin carried out the numerical part of the evaluation. They held the records of workshops and who attended them, and were able to monitor this on an ongoing basis, which enabled the reasons for any events such as cancellations or non-attendance to be more clearly identified.

Dave and Tamsin had each taken primary responsible for particular workshop groups, but held the final workshop with one another's groups, as they felt that the pupils might feel less constrained to give the 'right answers' or feel they were being tested with a different facilitator. They also planned to do this for the follow-up evaluation at six months. They had considered getting a third party to conduct the final discussions, but it was likely to be practically difficult to do this, and they felt that a third party might not fully understand the intentions of the workshops or evaluations, or give them the priority that they did.

The Ethics of the Evaluation

The evaluation of the workshops formed the natural conclusion of the project as a whole. Consent from head teachers, parents, and pupils had been secured for the entire project, and this included the evaluation phase. Ground rules regarding confidentiality, and situations where confidentiality would have to be breached (such as child protection issues), were set and agreed at the start of the workshops, and these were reiterated for the evaluation sessions. The pupils' actual names were altered for the evaluation report; however, participants were reminded that those who knew them well, particularly those who had been in their group, might recognise them in the report. The groups were reminded of their responsibilities to maintain the confidentiality of information given by, and identities of, others. Pupils were not obliged to participate in the evaluation, even if they had attended other workshops. All those who had participated were invited to be a part of the evaluation.

GUIDED WORK

This section revisits the learning outcomes covered in the chapter. You may want to complete it alone, or with colleagues.

1. Determine the right time to evaluate various elements of change.

Identify a change that you would like to make in practice.

- List the aim and objectives of this innovation.
- Make a plan for this innovation (you may wish to use the one you developed in the guided work in Chapter 4).
- On the plan, indicate when each stage could realistically be evaluated and why you have chosen this timescale for evaluation.

2. Understand a range of approaches to, and methods of, evaluating change.

Using the plan you have developed above:

- Describe what approach you would use to gather evaluative information at each stage and why this would be the best approach (for example, qualitative/quantitative/a mixture of approaches).
- Describe the methods you would use to gather evaluative information at each stage and why these would be suitable (for example, checklist/interview/discussion/observation/measurement).
- Think about what might influence the accuracy of the information gathered using each method.
- Consider whether these approaches and methods will also enable you to capture unexpected information and outcomes.
- Decide whether these methods will tell you whether change has happened, what the effect of it is, and enable you to ascertain why this was.

3. Select an appropriate way to interpret the information gathered in evaluation activities.

- Describe how you would analyse the information you gathered for each stage of the evaluation described above.
- Think about whether anything might affect the accuracy of your interpretation.
- If anything could affect the accuracy of your interpretation, how might you overcome it?

4. Appreciate the ethical issues involved in the evaluation of change.

Using the plan you developed above, for each stage of evaluation, consider:

- Who would be involved in the evaluation activities (for example, who would be observed, interviewed, have their work assessed)?
- How would you decide who would be involved?

- Would people have a choice over whether they were involved?
- What might their concerns be about the evaluation?
- How would you allay these concerns?
- What benefits would the evaluation bring?
- Could the evaluation have any adverse effects for individuals or groups?
- Do the benefits outweigh the risks of harm?

Additional Resources

http://changesuk.net/services/evaluation/

http://www.evaluationtrust.org/tools/introduction

http://www.evaluationtoolbox.net.au/index.php?option=com_content&view=article&id=40&Itemid=126

http://www.socialresearchmethods.net/kb/intreval.htm

http://www.ucl.ac.uk/public-engagement/research/toolkits/Methods

9

Change That Doesn't Work Out

Chapter Learning Outcomes

After studying this chapter, the reader will be able to:

- Identify why a change in practice may not meet its aim
- Consider possible positive outcomes from a change that has not achieved its original aim
- Plan how to feed back to those who have been involved in or affected by change projects that have not had the expected outcome.

Summary

This chapter discusses change that has not achieved its aim. It highlights the importance of identifying why a change did not end as planned, including considering whether the idea, method of implementation, timing, factors external to the change itself, or a combination of these, made the planned change problematic. It also explores the possible positive outcomes of a change that has not achieved its original aim, discusses the need to avoid blaming oneself or others for apparently unsuccessful change, and the process of feeding back to those who have been involved in or affected by change projects that have not had the expected outcome.

Naz works on a four-bed children's high dependency unit (HDU). The unit does not cater for children who require fully assisted ventilation, but can accept those who need Continuous Positive Airways Pressure (CPAP) or Bilevel Positive Airways Pressure (BiPAP). At least two of the unit beds are often occupied by children who require long-term CPAP or BiPAP, but who would not otherwise require high dependency care.

The unit policy had always been that parents can visit at any time, but are not permitted to sleep on the unit overnight. When the unit was set up it was agreed that the severity of the children's illnesses made it necessary to have good access around their bed spaces, and that having to wake sleeping parents in order to carry out urgent interventions could pose a risk. However, there are very few facilities for parents to stay outside the unit, and they often end up sleeping in chairs by their child's bed, which is not comfortable for them, and creates an obstruction for staff. The unit received several complaints from parents who were unable to stay, and whose children became distressed because of it. As a result of this, the unit staff were asked to think about ways in which they could address the issue of patents staying overnight. Naz suggested trialling parents being able to sleep on fold-up beds beside their children's beds in the way that they could on other wards on the children's unit. Her suggestion met with a mixed response, but the decision was taken by the unit team to trail this approach for six months. As it was her idea, Naz took the lead in implementing the trial of this way of working.

Although the consensus had been to try this approach, during the six month trial Naz often felt that no one actually agreed with it. There always seemed to be reasons why parents were not able to stay on the unit at night, and although many of these seemed plausible, at the end of the six months, parents still rarely stayed overnight and Naz had the distinct impression that the staff did not really want them to. Her formal evaluation of the project included noting, on a day-by-day basis over a four-week period, how many parents did stay overnight, and holding discussions with nursing staff and parents to gauge their views on the innovation. The statistics supported her impression that very few parents stayed. In her discussions with parents, Naz found that most would have liked to stay on the unit overnight, but did not think that this was possible. Many parents reported that they had been advised that they should leave the unit at night, and felt obliged to do so. Some parents said that they had been told that they needed to leave to get some rest, but others stated that they had been told they would be in the way if they stayed, or that them staying was against health and safety regulations. A number of parents said that they knew they could stay, but that the staff did not have time to find them a bed, or did not want them on the unit. A few parents preferred or needed to leave the unit at night, but those who had wanted to stay had seldom felt able to.

In her discussions with nursing staff, Naz was generally told that whilst in principle people agreed with the idea of parents being able to stay overnight, in practice this did not work. The reasons given included: there was not enough space; there were concerns for safety because it might be difficult to access children to administer urgent interventions with parents there; the doctors did not like it; there was not time to get beds set up for the parents;

and parents needed to leave the unit to get a break and some sleep. Two staff said that they did not think that parents should be permitted to stay, because they would be in the way, but most suggested that they supported the idea in principle, but found it difficult to uphold in practice. Because several nurses had suggested that the medical staff did not like parents to stay, Naz extended her evaluation to asking medical staff their views. Most medical staff said that they had no real preference for whether parents stayed or not, and one doctor said that she had twice asked parents if they would like to stay on the unit overnight, but had then found that the nurses did not like them to.

Overall, the evaluation suggested to Naz that the trial had not really changed anything, or resolved the situation regarding parents staying on the unit at night.

Not all attempts at innovation will go as planned, or succeed in meeting their aims.

Identifying Why Things Didn't Work

When you have attempted to change practice, but do not seem to have achieved your aim, it is useful to try to identify why this was: whether the aim of the innovation, the way the change was addressed or implemented, or something external to the change itself was the problem (Reid et al. 2007). This helps you to decide whether it is worth spending more time on trying to implement the new way of working, or whether you should simply move on because, at this point in time at least, it will not work.

The aim of Naz's project had been to enable those parents who wanted to sleep by their child's bed at night to do so, and her impression was that although there were some practical challenges to achieving this aim, the main issue was that there had never really been what Hall and Hord (2011: 219–224) and Cameron and Green (2009: 185) describe as a critical mass who had bought into the new way of working. Two other people had thought it was a good idea and offered to help her with the project, about three others had seemed in favour, two people had been strong opponents, but the majority had been fairly indifferent. She suspected that the views of the two opponents created a stronger force than the enthusiasm or agreement of the two or more supporters. This meant that, in terms of the driving and restraining forces created by staff, those restraining, or working against, change were greater than those driving it (Lewin 1951, Parkin 2009: 152–153).

The two staff who strongly opposed the idea of parents staying were not particularly senior staff, but both had worked on the children's unit for a long time, and were inclined to influence other staff. They were, therefore, opinion leaders and key players (Iles and Cranfield 2004, Richens et al. 2004). Naz felt that their opinions had remained unchanged throughout the project, and it was likely that no one on a shift with them would have felt confident to invite parents to stay if they opposed the idea. Although a couple of people had supported Naz's suggestion, they were probably not as influential as the two opponents, even though one of them was more senior. The general feeling of indifference from other staff would have meant that having to risk the disapprobation of opinion leaders would have easily swung things in favour of not adopting the new approach.

Unsuccessful Innovation: Was There a Critical Mass?

Whose idea was it?
How many people were strongly in favour of it?
What was their level of influence?
How many people were slightly in favour of it?
What was their level of influence?
How many people were strongly opposed to it?
What was their level of influence?
How many people were slightly opposed to it?
What was their level of influence?
How many people were indifferent to it?
Who would have influenced those who were indifferent?

Kyriakidou (2011) suggests that people may view a proposed change as either attractive or non-engaging, and if it is non-engaging, they may not really oppose it, but will probably not feel inclined to spend time and effort in participating. Naz felt that the staff on the unit probably mostly viewed parents staying overnight in this way, and were not opposed to, but were fairly indifferent about, it. Apathy can work very powerfully against change (Giangreco and Peccei 2005) as people are unlikely to make time, effort, or take any particular risk (including the risk of displeasing opinion leaders), to accommodate a new way of working in which they have no real interest. Naz felt that, as well as the views of opinion leaders, the overall lack of enthusiasm for parents staying on the unit at night probably meant that any practical barriers would have become significant restraining forces. The fold-up beds for parents to use had to be collected from a cupboard just outside the unit, and on a busy shift, Naz realised that the inconvenience of this arrangement could easily become a restraining force. Looking at her evaluation data, she saw that several parents had reported that the nurses: 'Said they would find me a bed but never did', so there seemed not to be so much a refusal to get beds for parents, as this simply not being enough of a priority for it to happen very often.

Opinion leaders, regardless of their level of seniority, can make or break whether an innovation succeeds or not.

In terms of readiness for change, Naz realised that most people on the unit were not actually ready to change their practice. At least two were at the stage of pre-contemplation (Prochaska and DiClemente1992), and did not see changing the way things were done as necessary or desirable. Most were probably at the stage of contemplation, thinking that parents staying by their child's bed might in principle be a good option, but were not completely convinced that it really was a good idea, or a priority. The majority of staff were therefore likely to still be weighing up the pros and cons of it, rather than strongly committed to changing the way they did things (Prochaska and DiClemente 1992). Very few were at the stage of determination to change, ready and willing to make a significant effort to alter the way things were done (Prochaska and DiClemente 1992). On reflection, Naz felt that enabling parents to stay on the unit overnight had not been achievable because she had introduced it before there were a sufficient number of people who were ready enough for change to counter balance the restraining force of those who were not yet ready to contemplate it. The restraining forces had never diminished, and the driving forces had not increased, and thus, change had not really been achievable.

In order to decide the next steps to take, Naz had to consider whether a critical mass that supported this initiative could be created, or whether the project should be shelved, or abandoned for the foreseeable future. She reviewed the way she had shared her ideas, and although she felt that there were some ways in which she could have improved this, she did not think this would ever have made a great difference. She had shared her idea at a meeting that was called because of complaints from parents about the problems that not being able to stay on the unit at night created for them and their children. No one else had made any suggestions, and thus her idea had been chosen by the group as the way forward: the team had endorsed this and suggested she lead it. As a staff nurse on the unit, she had not felt that the change in practice had been seen as imposed from above, but rather as a solution that had come from the frontline workforce: a bottom-up approach to change (Hall and Hord 2011: 12). On reflection, though, because the unit was required to address this issue because of complaints that had been made, she thought that perhaps the initiative could have been perceived as being imposed from the top down (Hall and Hord 2011: 15). Although the unit staff had been left to direct how they would address the issue, Naz felt that they probably did not generally feel ownership of the need for change, or of the innovation (Palmer 2004, Pare et al. 2011). It was more likely that they perceived the situation as being that something had to be seen to be done, and her idea would fulfil this. They had probably accepted that this would be a good way to be seen to be doing something, rather than buying in to actually doing it.

If an innovation has not worked out, it may be worth considering whether people agreed to try working in a new way, or agreed to 'be seen to be doing something.'

Naz wondered if things would have been different if she had accessed more support for her project from outside the HDU nursing team. She had seen this as mainly a nursing issue, as nurses were the ones who essentially acted as the gatekeepers of whether or not parents could stay overnight. Her manager had been happy for this innovation to be trialled, as a solution to the problem, but had not been particularly involved in or overtly supportive of it. Naz had accepted this, thinking it would enhance the innovation by it being seen as mainly owned as 'shop floor' level. However, she now considered whether if it would have been useful to have had more explicit support from her manager, and senior medical staff, such as the paediatrician who oversaw the unit. Although both had, in principle, agreed to the project, they had not really been involved with it, and the term 'not disagreed' might better describe their views and input. Having more upfront endorsement from them might have been an important counterbalance to the negative forces of those who opposed the idea. It might also have reduced the fear of the consequences of change (Grol and Grimashaw 2003). Concerns that having a parent by the bedside at night was unsafe might have been lessened by clarity over who had approved their presence.

When Naz looked at the timing of this change, there was no other significant project or new initiative in progress that was competing with it for time or resources (Palmer 2004, Golden 2006). Neither was it a particularly busy time for the unit as a whole, although the workload was cited by some nurses as a reason for being unable to get beds for parents (Oxman and Flottorp 2001, Grol and Grimashaw 2003). The process of getting beds for parents would often need to take place at the end of one shift or the start of the next, which were busy times. Given the lack of enthusiasm for the initiative, Naz wondered if reducing the effort required to get beds for parents might have made the new way of working more successful. If the HDU had fold-up beds pre-placed at each bed space, or beds that could fold down from the wall, then the initiative might have worked. It would also have been harder for staff to dissuade parents from staying if they saw a bed available. Looking back, Naz felt that she could have given more consideration to the practical and resources side of the trial (Hall and Hord 2011: 149–150). By allowing the situation to seem clumsy and temporary, without ideal resources, she thought that she might have inadvertently given the message that the plan was short term, and not expected to succeed. As she now felt that this was perhaps how most staff saw the initiative, the lack of resources might have reinforced this view.

Why Has Change not Succeeded?

Why was it introduced?
How were people told about it?
Who was involved in making the decision to attempt the innovation?
What evidence was there to support it?
Were the necessary resources in place?
Were enough people ready enough for change when it was rolled out?
Was this a priority for individuals or teams?
Was there managerial support for the change?
Was the aim achievable?
Was the timing problematic?
Were there any factors external to the change itself that might have worked against it?
Did those leading change seem to others to be committed to making the innovation work?

Although Naz identified some ways in which she could have changed how she introduced and resourced the new way of working, she felt that her main misjudgement had been assuming that the agreement to the trial would mean that people would make it an everyday priority. The reality seemed to be that most staff were not opposed to parents staying overnight, but did not see it as enough of a priority to make any great effort to enable it to happen. She thought that however much she tweaked the day-to-day project management processes, unless this core ethos changed, little progress would be made. Anderson, Klein and Stuart (2000) suggest that no change can occur without those involved substantively changing how they see things, and Naz concluded that this change in the way people viewed parents' staying on the unit at night had not occurred. Unless this happened, however much attention she gave to the rest of her action plan, it was unlikely to succeed.

Naz now thought that it might have been useful to have collected more evidence to support her idea (there was very limited evidence for or against her plans though) (Plastow 2006). Perhaps more importantly, she wondered if, instead of jumping in with ideas to solve the issue of parents being able to stay overnight, it would have been better for the unit team to have carried out a problem analysis of some kind (as described in Chapter 2). This would perhaps have enabled them to explore what the actual problems and root causes of the complaints received regarding parents staying overnight were. If the problem was that parents were unable to stay on the unit, the problem analysis process might have been a means of discussing this, and challenging people's views on the matter, so that solutions that addressed the causes of parents being unable to stay could be found. Equally, it might be that further exploration would have uncovered that the actual problem was not that parents were unable to stay by their child's bed, but that there was nowhere near the HDU where they could stay, or that the events surrounding their departure were problematic, rather than them actually wanting to sleep on the HDU itself. A problem analysis might also have uncovered that it was not expedient for parents to stay by their child's bed on HDU, and that the real issue was managing expectations, and providing greater clarity over what would and would not be possible for parents, and why.

After reviewing her action plan, and thinking about why the outcome had not been what she had hoped for, Naz concluded that at this point in time it was not worthwhile to continue to try to accommodate parents on the HDU at night. She felt that for progress to be made, a clearer analysis of the problem of parents being unable to stay on the unit overnight, and possible causes of this, was needed. This might, she thought, usefully include unit staff reflecting on what their views, attitudes, and priorities related to parents staying overnight were. Managing things in this way would have made the approach to change closer to a transformational approach to developing practice described in Chapter 1, where change is the result of critical reflection enabling individuals and teams to perceive things differently and to design new ways of working because of it (Dewing 2010, Walsh et al. 2011).

When an innovation doesn't work out: ask yourself if it was addressing the cause of a problem, or its effect.

Learning from Unsuccessful Change

If, after having apparently had instruction or support to change practice, and gone to some effort to do so, the new way of working does not go to plan, and practice does not change, it is very discouraging. However, although it does not feel like it just then, change that has not worked out, or has not gone to plan, can still be very important. Whilst it can feel as if this is unfair after all your efforts, the reality is that not all change succeeds in meeting its aims (Welch and McCarville 2003). Higgs and Rowland (2005) suggest that up to 70% of change initiatives fall into this category. This does not mean that change in general is not worth trying, or that something not working as it was hoped it would is always a failure. Many changes in practice are attempted because someone wonders if something would work, and if you have evidence from your efforts that it does not, it can stop you and other people from wasting time and effort in thinking about it again. There had been debate since the paediatric HDU opened about whether or not to let parents stay on the unit at night. If, after everything else had been considered, the final consensus decision from the trial turned out to be that this was not feasible, staff could avoid devoting any more time to wondering about it, or trying it out. The answer to whether something will work or not can legitimately go either way, and a project that asks, 'Will this work?' has to be able to accept either yes or no as the answer.

It is also often possible to learn useful things about the organisation and those in it from unsuccessful change. In this instance, one of the things that Naz felt had become clear was that whilst the organisation as whole subscribed to the principles of involving parents in their child's care, and partnership with parents, the paediatric HDU did not really have the resources, space, or ethos, required to make parents being able to sleep on the unit a reality. In future projects, she felt that she would begin any attempt at innovation by spending more time reflecting on her own views, values, priorities, and assumptions, and exploring those of other team members, before trying to alter the way things were done.

Despite feeling that her efforts had been largely wasted, Naz had now identified, from rereading the initial complaints, and from her discussions with parents, that the parents who had complained, and those who were most unhappy about not being able to stay at night, were those whose children needed long-term CPAP or BiPAP. This led her to consider whether the unit had, in fact, been trying to address the right problem.

Change is an experiment with a new way of working: it may or may not have the expected result.

Unsuccessful Change and Unexpected Positive Outcomes

Change that has not resulted in the expected outcome is often seen as unsuccessful. There may, however, be unexpected outcomes from a change, which can include positive things (Higgs and Rowland 2005). One of the unexpected outcomes of Naz's work was that it highlighted the question of whether HDU was really the right place for children who always needed

CPAP or BiPAP, and were admitted to hospital for other reasons, which would not of themselves merit HDU admission. This was an ongoing debate, and Naz's work showed that being unable to stay with their children overnight on HDU was more problematic for the parents or carers of this group of children than for others. Her evaluation data indicated that some of these children struggled to communicate without their parents or carers there, and that they were often on HDU longer than the average child, so having no one to stay with them overnight posed additional challenges for them. Because these children were generally clinically stable, albeit requiring long-term respiratory support, they were also less likely than others to require unexpected interventions, which parental presence at the bedside might impede. One outcome from Naz's attempted innovation was that it added the final ammunition to an ongoing debate about where children who had this type of need should be accommodated. This resulted in a commitment by the Trust to establish a two-bed area, which would take children who required any form of long-term-assisted ventilation. This was ostensibly nothing to do with Naz's initial project's aims, but it was a useful development and would mean that in the area designated for this purpose, children's parents would be able to stay with them at night.

Recalling what prompted a change in practice may help to clarify whether or not an apparent 'failure' is in fact what it seems. The issue of parents being able to stay overnight had mainly been highlighted because of complaints from the parents of children who needed long-term CPAP or BiPAP. The project had potentially led to a development in services that would enable this group of parents to stay. So, in terms of achieving something useful, the project had contributed to resolving the problem that had initiated its development, even though it had not met its own stated aims.

Innovations that Don't Work Can Still Be Used to Develop Practice

They can provide direction about what should or should not be attempted in future

They can provide insights into organisational culture and priorities

They can make teams and individuals re-evaluate the original problem

They can have useful spin-offs that positively influence practice

If change is about improving practice, then knowing that your project influenced this in some way is important, even if the direction of influence was not exactly what you planned. In Naz's case, the children in question represented a significant amount of the HDU workload, so their being better accommodated and being able to have their parents to stay with them was an important development in their care provision. It would also free up HDU beds for other acute work. So, this benefit of the project having run was worth noting, even though its aim had not been achieved.

Change that does not go to plan can still have useful outcomes.

Planning New Directions

An important part of any change in practice is planning what to do once the stage of the project that you planned is complete. This is equally important when the planned change has not worked out. A part of planning what to do next is identifying what did not work and why. Sometimes a project will have shown that a new way of working does not work, and that the best thing to do is to abandon it and go back to the previous way of working: if something really is not a good idea then it is quite right to stop trying to do it. It may, however, be that the unexpected outcomes from a change project become the focus of ongoing work. The new project that arose, at least in part, from Naz's work was establishing the long-term ventilation unit. Whilst this was a spin-off from the original plan, it was an important development. It would also allow the HDU staff the chance to determine whether the issue of parents wanting to stay overnight still existed with a slightly different client group.

Although it may be entirely appropriate to abandon a change that has not gone to plan, it is worth thinking about why you tried the new approach before completely moving away from it. If the change was instigated because of a problem in practice, then you may need to look at alternatives, because the problem that initiated it may not have gone away even if that solution did not work. Naz had instigated the new way of working because parents, particularly those whose children needed long-term BiPAP or CPAP, had complained about being unable to stay on the unit overnight. Although the children who required long-term CPAP or BiPAP might now be better catered for, the problem might still exist for other children and families. If parents continued to express a desire to stay at night, then Naz felt that alternative approaches would need to be explored.

Feeding Back

Feeding back to those who have participated in change is important, however, this can be harder when things have not gone to plan, because there is not an upbeat message of success to share. Nonetheless, because things will have been learned, and the direction that the team or teams involved now need to take needs to be clear, feedback is important. If the project is being abandoned, those involved need to know this, and if something else is being tried, or the project tweaked, or suspended for now, this also needs to be made known.

One of the key features of feeding back following a project that has not worked out is to avoid blame. When all your efforts have come to nothing, it is natural and easy to want to blame someone or something. However, whilst it is a good idea to try to identify why things have not worked out, blaming anyone, including yourself, for long, is not helpful. Looking at why things went wrong, and what might have helped the change to work, is important, but it is more useful to highlight issues than individuals. If people have deliberately sabotaged a new way of working, blaming them will only highlight their success. In Naz's case, she was fairly sure that the two people who had always opposed her project had been instrumental in its failure. However, as they had consistently stated that they did not agree with the project, to complain that they were the cause of its downfall would be pointless and only illustrate that they were either right or had the power to sabotage efforts at change. If people have been trying to subtly sabotage your project, highlighting that it is their fault may be tempting, because you may feel that others should know what they have done, or see how they were taken in by them, but it has exactly the same effect as blaming people who openly sabotage your work. Naz had been slightly annoyed that some members of staff who had apparently supported her idea and agreed to promote it had then not followed this up by doing as they promised very effectively. Nonetheless, rather than questioning them personally, at the feedback meeting where the outcomes of the project were discussed, she explained that whilst some people had been enthusiastic about the project when it was suggested, and the unit as a whole had agreed to trial it, the evaluation suggested that no one had really found they could carry through its principles day to day. This meant that she did not blame anyone, but subtly reminded those who had agreed to participate of their joint ownership of the decision, and clarified that the initiative had been a shared venture, which had not shown a clear way forward in resolving the issue that precipitated it. It also gave her a chance to ask the group as a whole to look at why the venture had not succeeded. This meant that the discussion was not a personal dispute, but a chance to debate shared values, which was the main issue, Naz felt, for any ongoing decisions about whether or not to attempt to enable parents to stay on the unit overnight. The majority of staff owned that whilst they did not mind parents staying on the unit, it was problematic in reality, and that they did not feel strongly enough in favour of it for organising the practicalities to take priority over other aspects of their work. There were also concerns that the unit was no big enough to safely accommodate parents at night. From this, the team were able to agree that they might request that a small area near the unit be considered for conversion to an area for parents to stay, rather than reattempting bedside accommodation, which people now felt able to admit they did not really support. Whilst Naz was irritated that no one had said this before, she felt that at least now there was a realistic and honest statement of intent and commitment. It also confirmed her own reflections about why this innovation had not worked.

If there are positive outcomes from a change that has not gone to plan, then these should be emphasised as a part of feeding back. Naz highlighted that this project had enabled the Trust to look in more detail at who was using HDU beds and seek a new way of providing for children who needed long-term-assisted ventilation. As well as giving a positive message, it meant that if Naz later tried to introduce another change, she could recall this project as being the one from which the long-term ventilation unit was established, rather than as the one that did not work.

All those who have been involved in an attempt to change practice should be aware of its outcomes (Hall and Hord 2011: 154). In Naz's case, this was mainly the nursing staff, but as some nurses had suggested that medical staff did not want parents to stay, she invited both nursing and medical staff to the feedback meeting. As not everyone could attend the meeting, she sent an email summary to all staff, and placed a note in the communication book. She also met with the unit manager, to put forward the new proposal, before making the communications about the meeting public. Naz considered how to give feedback to parents who had participated in the project: as they had given time to share their views, she felt that they had a right to know the outcome, and what to expect in future if their children needed another HDU admission. However, to write to each parent would be difficult, so she decided to make expectations clearer for current and future parents by displaying a poster about the trial prominently, where parents could easily read it. This addressed one of the issues that remained at the end of the project, about managing expectations for staff and parents, and clarifying to parents why overnight accommodation on the unit was not available at present, and what was being done to try to address this.

Providing feedback is as important when change has not been successful in achieving its aim as when it has been.

Summary

Although change that does not go to plan, or achieve its aims, is discouraging for those who have invested time and energy in it, as much, and sometimes more, can be learned from things that do not work out as planned as from those that do. When change does not work out, it is useful to consider why this was, and whether the idea, method of implementation, timing, another factor or factors, or a combination of these, made the planned change problematic. It can also be useful to think about whether the way in which the new way of working was planned allowed the things that might contribute to its success or otherwise to be identified, including the views, values, priorities and assumptions of those involved.

It is important to feed back to those involved on the outcomes of all innovations, and this is equally important when change has not gone to plan or had the expected outcomes, so that everyone knows what has happened, and what the plans for the future are.

Key Points

If change does not achieve its expected aim, it is useful to see if you can identify why this was.

An innovation that does not achieve its original aim can still have positive outcomes.

Providing feedback is as important when change has not gone to plan as when it has.

CASE STUDY

Debra works on an acute medical admissions ward. Some of the patients who are admitted to the ward border on being critically ill, and should ideally be housed on an HDU or CCU. However, the pressure on acute beds, particularly during the winter months, means that they can often only be accommodated on the medical admissions ward. This group of patients often need additional observations or interventions, and more fluid management, than the charts that the ward uses can easily accommodate. This became problematic for staff, who felt that they were constantly trying to tweak the existing charts, and that the result was a very crowded and difficult to read record of events, which did not give a very clear picture of the patient's clinical condition, or what interventions they had received.

Because of this, a new chart was designed for use with the more highly dependent patients. It was initially used regularly, no major problems were encountered in its use, and medical and nursing staff generally commented favourably on it. However, over time it gradually stopped being used, and people returned to adapting the standard charts for the more highly dependent patients.

How Was the Decision to Make the Change Reached?

When the ward team explored the options to address the problem they were having with charting information about the more seriously ill patients, the favoured suggestion was to design specific observation and fluid charts for use with patients who required a higher than usual level of monitoring or intervention. Debra volunteered to lead in the design and implementation of these charts. She worked on this with two middle grade medical staff, and two other nurses.

Was the Aim Achievable?

- The aim of this initiative was to provide a means of easily but accurately recording the clinical condition and therapies provided to patients who were deemed to need more interventions than the standard observation and fluid charts catered for. The objectives were to provide one chart which could be used to record a patient's heart rate, blood pressure, temperature, respiratory rate, central venous pressure, Glasgow coma score, pain score, oxygen saturation level, percentage of oxygen received, and cardiac rhythm, half hourly for 12 hours.
- to provide one chart that could be used to record up to eight fluid infusions, and fluid outputs, hourly, for a 12 hour period.

Debra thought that this aim had been achievable, as the form was designed, piloted, and considered to be fit for purpose. However, on reflection she thought that whilst the aim and objectives had been achieved, there had been no objective, and thus less attention given to, the circumstances in which the charts should be used.

Did People Know Why the Change Was Being Requested?

The new charts were developed as a result of a problem highlighted by medical and nursing staff on the ward. The development of the new charts was agreed at a ward meeting. Information about this decision was recorded in the ward communication book, emailed to medical and nursing staff, and restated at subsequent ward meetings, until and after the launch of the new charts. As far as Debra could tell, all the staff who would be using the charts had known that they were being designed, and why.

Did Enough People Support the Change?

Debra had been under the impression that almost all the ward staff supported the idea of a specific chart for use with the patients who required the most interventions. In terms of driving and restraining forces, the apparent weight of opinion was behind the change, with several staff seeming enthusiastic, a number agreeing, and only three who were not convinced. Even those three did not seem to oppose the idea. They simply did not see it as particularly necessary. They were not really opinion leaders on the ward, and the main opinion leaders seemed to Debra to favour the development of the chart. The more senior staff were also in favour of developing it. The medical staff generally seemed in favour of a specific chart being used for patients who required additional monitoring or interventions. Thus, there seemed to Debra to have been a strong enough driving force to merit developing the chart, with some hope of success.

Were the Necessary Resources Available?

The required resources were time to develop and pilot the charts, which Debra felt had been available, and resources for obtaining an ongoing supply of charts. A constant stock of about 100 charts was kept, with more ordered as stocks dwindled. Debra was not aware that stocks had ever run out, which would have created a need to return to adapting the standard charts.

Was There Frontline Support for the Change?

Not everyone from the ward was at the meeting where the decision to develop and use the charts was made, however, there was generally support for the idea and it had seemed to Debra that the majority of staff were either ready for this change, or at least (in the case of the staff who did not see the need for a new chart) willing to contemplate change. There was very little evidence of people being at the pre-contemplation stage. When the chart was piloted, although a few minor tweaks were required, there was no significant criticism, suggestion that the charts were not needed, or requests to abandon the initiative. The chart was initially used well, and the impression Debra had at the time was that the innovation was accepted, and most people changed their practice.

Was There Managerial Support or the Change?

Debra's manager had been happy for the change to go ahead. She had seen it as a good solution to the problem, but as it was a day-to-day clinical issue, she had not felt any need to be particularly involved in the innovation.

Did Anything in the Method of Implementing Change Detract from It Being Achieved?

Debra wondered if the charts had been interpreted as a solution to the seasonal variation in patient acuity, rather than being a new initiative to use with any highly dependent patient, at any time of the year. In the early days of the new charts being used, Debra had found that several staff were not sure if a particular patient was sick enough to merit using the new charts. These two issues led her to wonder if she could have clarified which patients the new chart was designed to be used for. She also wondered if some practicalities had detracted from the use of the new charts being sustained. The ward receptionist made up admission packs, which were ready to use as soon as a patient was admitted. However, these had not included the new charts. On busy shifts, although in principle everyone agreed to their value, having to find a chart to add to the admission pack might have meant that they were not always used. It might also have suggested that they were for occasional or seasonal use only, rather than regular and ongoing use with a specific patient group. Debra felt that perhaps it would have been useful to have had two types of admission pack, one standard and one for more seriously ill patients, for ease of use and clarity of purpose.

Was the Timing of Change Problematic?

Although the new charts were introduced when the ward was busy, and housed a relatively high number of very sick patients, this meant that they were needed, and immediately used. Debra felt that the challenge in terms of timing might have related more to the sustained use of the new charts. The charts were introduced in November, and for the first three months were used regularly. However, the time when less critically ill patients began to be admitted to the ward coincided with a time when it would be natural for any interest in a new initiative to wane, some three or so months after it was introduced. Debra felt that this was probably why use of the new charts had not been sustained. Their use was not yet established when the demand for them lessened for a period of time, and she and the team who assisted in developing them had not done anything to maintain their use other than occasionally ask people why they were not using them.

Debra realised that her evaluation of the new charts, and attempts to maintain their use, had been fairly casual. She was fairly sure that they had improved the recording of patients' conditions and events, and made the work of caring for very sick patients easier for nursing and medical staff. However, because she had not conducted a formal evaluation, she did not have any concrete evidence to promote their continued use, or any particular reason to remind people to use them. She now thought that a more formal evaluation might have been useful, and served to remind people of the existence of the charts, and their value. It could also have highlighted any issues or problems in their use, which could then have been addressed.

Were There any Factors External to the Change Itself that Might Have Worked against It?

There were no external factors, other than patient numbers, that Debra could think of which had influenced this change in practice. No other major changes were underway, and staffing levels were typical for the ward. There had been no significant staff turnover, which might have meant that people did not know about the new charts.

What Happened as a Result of the Attempt to Change Practice?

Initially, the new charts were used, and they appeared to fulfil their purpose of simplifying the recording of information and making it easier to see patient trends over a day at a glance. It was likely that this improved patient care. However, because of the lack of formal evaluation, Debra could not say with any certainty exactly what had happened because of the initiative, for good or bad.

The lack of sustained use of the charts, along with a resurgence of complaints about the inadequacy of the standard charts as the winter pressure on beds resumed, led Debra to question exactly what the problem that had presented as a need for a different chart was. The key issue seemed to be that there were patients on the ward whose acuity of illness exceeded, that which the ward was designed to cater for, and that as a result of this the standard charts were not adequate for their needs. There might also be an element of staff not being comfortable with caring for patients who were very seriously ill. In terms of identifying exactly what the problem was, it seemed to Debra that it was the level of acuity of some patient's illness that was a key factor, rather than charts per se, although they were a presenting feature of the issue.

This, alongside the occasional queries that Debra had received over when to use the new charts led her to consider whether the problem that needed to be addressed was the core remit of the ward, and perhaps greater clarity over when they were receiving patients who fell outside this. This would provide a clearer signal for when to use the new charts, and might at the same time be useful in establishing when the ward was functioning over and above its expected remit.

How Was Information on the Outcomes of the Project Fed Back?

Debra spoke at a ward meeting about the difficulties in using the standard charts for very sick patients seeming to have recurred. She reminded staff that a new chart had been introduced, which had been intended to address this issue, and that whilst it had originally worked well, it had slowly been abandoned. She invited feedback on this and, as she had suspected would be the case, most people recalled the chart, said they had liked it, and asked one another why they had stopped using it. It seemed to have simply slipped off their radar, and when a very sick patient came in was not a time when they were likely to recall it or to have time to look for one.

Debra suggested that as the problem of the inadequacy of the standard charts had resurfaced, they should perhaps explore the cause of the problem. Although she did not carry out a formal problem analysis, Debra encouraged staff to discuss what caused the need for charts to be altered. From this, they identified that the problem seemed to be that staff were dealing with patients outside the limits that the ward had been designed for. Debra suggested that rather than simply reintroducing the new charts, to patch up the problem during the winter months, they should determine, with appropriate liaison, what was and was not outside the standard ward remit. This would provide a forum for discussion of whether there were other options for housing very sick patients when HDU and CCU were full, and create greater clarity over what was expected of the medical admissions ward, and the staff who worked there. This in turn might provide an opportunity for discussing staffing levels and additional training or experience if staff did not feel confident in caring for the sicker patients. They could also develop or reintroduce the new charts, tying these to the definitions agreed on, and create two admission packs: one for standard admissions and one for higher dependency admissions. This would give greater clarity over when to use the new charts, make them readily available, and provide a reminder to use them.

The ward staff agreed that this would be a useful approach. Several staff felt that nothing would be done about staffing levels, training, or alternative locations for patients who fell outside the acute medical admissions ward remit. However, there was consensus that placing all these issues 'on the table' and highlighting to managerial levels that there was more than a need for a new chart was a positive development. There was also general support for the reintroduction of the charts, with new admission packs to aid the process.

In this way, Debra aimed to create not only renewed interest, but also corporate ownership of and commitment to, the new charts. She also felt that she had now sought to address the cause, not just the effect, of the problem.

Whilst reminding people of joint ownership and responsibility, she hoped that she had avoided suggesting blame for the cessation of chart usage.

Were There Positive Outcomes?

The positive outcomes from the new charts ceasing to be used were that, in addition to the ward team restating their value, and finding more user friendly ways to sustain their use, they had questioned what the problem that precipitated the chart adaptation was. This meant that the solution might more effectively address the cause, as well as the effect, of the problem. This might in turn mean that, in the longer term, the way that the more seriously ill patients were catered for, and how the staff on the medical admissions ward were equipped to care for them, was improved.

GUIDED WORK

This section revisits the learning outcomes covered in the chapter. You may want to complete it alone, or with colleagues.

1. Identify why a change in practice may not meet its aim.

Identify a change in practice that you have been involved in, or know about, which did not achieve its aim. Think about the possible reasons for this. You might include

- Why it was introduced?
- How people were told about it?
- Who was involved in designing the innovation?
- What evidence there was to support it?
- Whether the aim was achievable?
- Whether the necessary resources were in place?
- Whether enough people were ready enough to support the innovation when it was rolled out?
- Whether this was a priority for individuals or teams?
- Whether there was managerial support for the innovation?
- Whether the timing of the change was problematic?
- Whether there were any factors external to the change itself that might have worked against it?

2. Consider possible positive outcomes from a change that has not achieved its original aim.

Consider whether there were any positive outcomes from the attempt to change practice outline above. You might consider, for example:

- Whether it provided an answer to a question that had been asked for some time.
- Whether it led to any alternative, useful, innovations.
- Whether it provided insight into the team or organisation's culture and priorities.
- Whether it provided clarity over what could realistically be achieved.
- Whether it led to a re-evaluation of the original reason for the innovation.

3. Plan how to feed back to those who have been involved in or affected by change projects that have not had the expected outcome.

Imagine that you are responsible for telling the team involved in the innovation above about the project's ending.

- Who would you inform of the outcome of the project?
- What information would you give about the project's outcome?
- How would you explain the reason for the project not meeting its aim?
- How would you tailor this information for different groups?
- What message would you give about the next steps that would be taken?
- What positive messages would you give?

Additional Resources

http://www.cfar.com/Documents/KeyFactorsChange.pdf

http://theses.flinders.edu.au/uploads/approved/adt-SFU20060130.095828/public/01front.pdf

10

Maintaining Change

Chapter Learning Outcomes

After studying this chapter, the reader will be able to:

- Identify factors that will assist in sustaining change
- Appreciate the significance of continued post-innovation evaluation and feedback in sustaining change
- Perceive the importance of continued practice developments in sustaining new ways of working.

Summary

Although planning and implementing change requires considerable effort, equal attention should be given to how new practice will be maintained after the initial implementation. This chapter suggests some approaches to sustaining new practice and discusses ways of maintaining enthusiasm for, and commitment to, a new way of working. These include continued evaluation and feedback, planning ongoing practice development, keeping people informed of developments, and disseminating information about the new way of working.

Laura works on an orthopaedic ward where a number of patients have pre-existing self-care problems, and require assistance with eating and drinking. Some time ago, the ward received two complaints about patients not receiving enough help to enable them to eat and drink, and Laura had become aware that, with busy workloads, people sometimes did not get all the help they needed at mealtimes. Along with a small group of colleagues, she devised an adjustment to the patients' initial assessment document to highlight what they needed assistance with at mealtimes: for example, a cup to be placed near them, help with cutting up their food. A section was also added to the care plans detailing what help people needed with eating and drinking. Those who needed assistance at mealtimes had a green sticker placed on the documentation at the end of their beds, so that staff could be reminded at a glance about who needed help of some form at mealtimes.

The staff on Laura's ward varied in their enthusiasm for her idea. Some were very enthusiastic about it: Laura asked them to take on various roles in the project, and they effectively acted as change champions. The majority did not oppose the idea, but equally did not show great enthusiasm for it. They felt that there was no harm in doing this, as it did not present a great change to the assessment process, but they were not completely convinced of its necessity or value. Several staff felt that documentation and stickers would make no difference at all to whether or not people received assistance at mealtimes, as time and other priorities were the issue. Laura agreed that the problem was heavy workloads and other priorities. However, she explained that the idea behind the initiative was to act as a reminder to people who had many competing priorities, and to help in situations where staff from other wards were sent to help at mealtimes, as they could be asked to check on people with green stickers on their bedside documentation. She explained that their ward, along with the rest of the NHS Trust, were required to demonstrate that nutritional standards were being met, and that the new system would go some way towards demonstrating this, and show that they had responded to a criticism. It would also provide evidence about whether their staffing level was adequate for the number of patients requiring mealtime help, as she had arranged for the 'green sticker status' to be added to the ward dependency scores.

The initiative was implemented, and initially worked well. Now Laura wanted to make sure that it was sustained.

Risk of Regression

Although the initial implementation of an innovation is where the focus often is, effort is also required to sustain change over time, and enable it to become embedded in practice (Virani et al. 2009). Laura had done a good job of convincing people to adopt the mealtime initiative, and the initial evaluation indicated that it had led to better provision for patients who needed mealtime assistance. However, she knew that she would need to keep working on it to maintain this as a meaningful part of assessment, which was acted on.

When you are planning and rolling out change, your attention and energy, and that of your supporters, is on the project. Once the new way of working has been implemented, especially if it seems to be going well, it is very easy to take your eye off the ball and for what was successful change to slowly flounder and fade. This is a much more common reason for developments in practice to fail over time than initiatives being consciously stopped (Morrow et al. 2010). As time goes on, other priorities come along and, because everyone's attention has moved, unless the new way of working is very firmly established, people stop making an effort, things slowly return to exactly how they were before the change was instigated, and all your hard work is undone (Virani et al. 2009, Balasubramanian et al. 2010). Laura was aware that, as time went by, people might gradually begin to complete the assessment forms and care plans less diligently, not use the stickers, and, over time, everything would be exactly how it was before the innovation was introduced. She knew that, if the mealtime innovation was to be maintained, she needed to continue to focus her efforts on it after its apparently successful implementation.

Until a new way of working becomes what everyone automatically does, or 'refreezing' for everyone in Lewin's (1951) terms has occurred, those who have never accepted change can still convince others to revert to how things were. Unless a significant force of people continuing to engage in and promote the new way of working, any opposition can eat away at the support it has, and what was a success becomes a change that did not work out. Laura was aware that although she appeared to have convinced most people of the need for the new approach to managing mealtime assistance, there were still some people who regarded the initiative as a waste of time. Although they appeared to be in the minority, they could, overtly or covertly, discourage others people from completing the documentation and using the stickers, and slowly erode the apparent success of the project, especially as many people had been quite indifferent to it. Chapter 4 identified that some people may not accept change until it has become the new routine or standard practice. So, unless efforts are made to sustain change until it has reached this stage, it may still not be fully adopted (Virani et al. 2009).

One of Laura's strategies was to avoid thinking, or letting others think, that she have achieved her goal once her initiative had been rolled out and apparently adopted (Kotter 1995). Whilst it is always important to give encouragement, praise and a sense of progress and achievement, giving the impression that everything has been achieved too soon can mean that people stop making an effort before things are really established. Laura felt that if people saw the project as completed and established too early on, efforts to work in the new way would be relaxed and occasionally assessment or care plan entries would be missed, and stickers forgotten. This might create a slow drift back to previous practice. In addition, if people really want to stop change, they can use an early sense of achievement and task accomplished to encourage other to think that as the new way of working is established, no real effort needs to be made any more. Once everyone if off guard, anyone seeking to detract from the change can slowly but continuously drip feed the message that the new way of working can occasionally be neglected, or does not really work all the time. Gradually the successful change in practice will be eroded and people will, inadvertently, revert to a previous way of working (Kotter 1995). If anyone on Laura's ward was making an effort to stop the mealtimes initiative, they could encourage others to think that now that the new documentation and use of the stickers was established, it was occasionally acceptable, especially when they were busy, to miss out on the odd sticker, or care plan entry. Over time, more and more might be 'occasionally missed', and the re-established norm would be to omit the part of the assessment and care plan that had been added, and not to use the stickers.

Once Change Has Been Rolled Out, and Seems to Have Been Successful:

Watch out for a slow drift away from the new way of working.
Be alert to people thinking they can revert to the old way of working 'just once.'
Be aware of those who have not yet accepted change: they can still persuade others to join them.
When the next project or initiative comes along, make an extra effort to ensure that your innovation is not forgotten.

So, despite the understandable desire to celebrate success, and the importance of thanking everyone for their hard work, it may be better to mark the rolling out and initial adoption of the new way of working, whilst also keeping the impetus going by clarifying that the project still requires input and effort. Two weeks after the new way of documenting mealtime needs was rolled out, Laura fed back at a ward meeting, sent emails, and placed a note in the communication book thanking everyone for their hard work. She not only shared the results from her initial evaluation of how often the new forms and stickers were used, and with what apparent effect, but also clarified that she would monitor the project over the next few months, as this would enable her to see how things where at times when the ward faced different challenges. This gave the message that whilst she was pleased with the support she had had, and with the outcomes of the initiative so far, she was keeping an eye on things, and her efforts were not relaxing.

Even when change has been successfully implemented, it can still fail if people go back to doing things in the old way.

Planning and Action to Sustain Change

Any practical plans that are made for change should incorporate strategies for maintaining it (Golden 2006). This includes the supplies needed to work in a new way remaining available long term (Hagedorn et al. 2006). If supplies become scarce, it will not be long before someone finds the old supplies and uses those. A one-off return to the old way of doing things will afford those who do not like the new way of working the perfect opportunity to remind people of how easy and effective the old order was, and to raise doubts as to the benefit of the new system. Laura was aware that if the meal-time assistance stickers ran into short supply, or if people were obliged to use the old admission documentation, her project could easily be undermined. In addition to people being able to be persuaded that the old format really was better, it would give those who opposed the initiative the chance to list this as one more change, which had not been thought through and which lacked the necessary resources to sustain it.

Ongoing funding for any new initiative also needs to be considered (Virani et al. 2009). In your enthusiasm to secure the necessary financial support for a project to go ahead, it can be tempting, and indeed necessary, to accept funding for a pilot with no guarantee of ongoing resources. You may have no choice but to do this if long-term funding is not available, and if the outcome of the pilot phase is unknown ongoing funding may not be offered at the outset. However, as things progress, it is important to think about how you will keep new practice solvent. If there are not enough staff, or resources, for it to continue, it may have to be abandoned altogether. Equally, it may become less easy to manage, staff time be more stretched, practicalities may become more challenging, and it may slowly become unworkable or sufficiently difficult that people begin to abandon it. Laura's work did not really require any specific resources other than the stickers. However, an agreement had been made, which she had shared with her colleagues, that the 'green sticker' status would contribute to the ward dependency scoring system. It was important that this agreement, and the resources which it demanded in terms of additional staff, continued to be acted to over time. Otherwise, one of the reasons why people had bought into change would be eroded, and with it, potentially, their support.

Ongoing education and training to sustain and develop new practice also merits consideration when you are planning change (Virani et al. 2009, Hall and Hord 2011: 150). Although Laura's initiative did not require staff to undergo any specific training, she wanted to be sure that any staff who joined the ward team knew about the system, why it existed, and how to use it. She considered it important that new staff induction programs had time ring fenced for this, and initially she wanted herself or one of her change champions to provide this input. Otherwise, it might fall to someone who was not really convinced about the value of the system. This meant that she needed to make sure that she or one of the change champions was available for a short slot in all staff inductions. Otherwise, new staff might not get the right message, or might get no particular message, and, over time, there was a risk that the system would fade and fail because a critical mass of staff were no longer aware of its existence.

In Chapter 5, the need to acknowledge and support the losses that change can bring was highlighted (Austin and Currie 2003, Scott et al. 2003, Price 2008, Hall and Hord 2011: 84). As a new way of working continues, and becomes established, thinking about and addressing feelings of loss remains important (Golden 2006). Losses may become less acceptable, rather than diminishing, as time goes on and people may encounter losses that they had not anticipated. Those who had hoped that a project would never work may realise that it is succeeding, and that the losses they thought they would avoid are becoming real. At the same time, aspects of the innovation that people had not really considered may begin to cause them to feel loss. At the outset of the mealtime initiative, Laura had been aware that one of the healthcare assistants felt that she had always done a very good job of making sure everyone knew who needed help with eating and drinking, reminding staff about this, and making sure that she checked on all the patients who needed help. Laura had seen that there was the potential for her role to be eroded by the mealtime initiative, and had therefore invited this member of staff to take a lead role in the new way of working, so that she still had a key role in guiding people about mealtime assistance. However, there was a possibility that her lead role would diminish as the new way of working became embedded as routine practice, and that she would begin to feel a loss of position. Laura tried to build in ways to keep this person's role central, including involving her in the evaluation activities, in the orientation of new staff, and providing formal feedback to staff, so that she continued to have, and be seen to have, a lead role, even as the day to day input required of her diminished.

It is also important to make sure that any benefits that staff have been promised from an innovation materialise. Change is generally easier to implement if those leading it are seen as trustworthy (Golden 2006), and sustaining change is likely to be more successful if people see those instigating it as trustworthy, and that any promises that were made are perceived to have been kept. If people have participated in change because of what they think they will gain from it, but do not derive the expected benefits, they are likely to become discontented and begin to withdraw support for the new way of working. One of the potential benefits of the new way of documenting mealtime needs had been that staff could use the number of patients who required green stickers to give tangible evidence of their mealtime work-load. However, for this to be meaningful, it had to have a direct outcome. Although green sticker use was included on the dependency forms, Laura negotiated about what could be done to assist the ward when they reached a critical level of green stickers. An agreement was reached that at a level of ten green stickers, the ward would need an extra staff member at mealtimes, unless they already had additional staffing above their established numbers. Laura was still aware that for this to positively influence staff views, it had to be acted on, and her role included reminding those organising staffing of the agreement that had been made. This did not always meet with success, but someone was often sent to assist, and her colleagues at least knew that she was keeping her part of the deal, and reminding others of the agreement that had been made.

After Change Has Been Rolled Out:

Make sure that the resources it requires remain available.
Be alert to losses that people may feel as it becomes more established.
Ensure that any promised benefits materialise.
Continue to feed back to all those involved.
Keep people up to date with any developments.
Create opportunities for new staff to learn about it.

Ongoing Evaluation

A part of maintaining change is checking that it is still happening, and achieving its aim, well after it has been introduced. Carrying out ongoing evaluation, far beyond the end of the original implementation, can help you to know whether or not this is so. Laura planned evaluations at dif-ferent stages after implementation of the mealtime initiative. The first was planned to take place a week after the new paperwork had been introduced (to find out whether things had actually happened as planned), the second a month after the new way of working was introduced (to see how the new documentation and stickers were bedding down, and their effects), a third at six months after implementation (to see if the momentum for change was sustained), and the fourth one year after the change was rolled out (to see whether, over time, the new way of working really was established).

This frequency and duration of formal evaluation enabled Laura to check on the effectiveness of the innovation over a whole year, so as to capture potential challenges posed by changing workloads at different times. It also meant that she could detect early warning signs of any return to previous practice, and make the point that the new way of working was still on her radar, and would continue to be monitored. If things were going well, she could continue to provide positive feedback and reinforcement to give people the incentive to keep going. If things were slipping, she could provide reminders, and explore what the problems with maintaining the mealtime initiative were. Once the stimulus for change is gone, interest in it may diminish, and without reminders of why it was introduced, as improvements become the new norm, the problems that led to innovation can be forgotten (Virani et al. 2009). Laura wanted to use the chance to feed back from evaluations as an opportunity to remind people where they had come from, and where they were now, so that the benefits of the new way of working remained clear.

The way in which you plan evaluation over the longer term needs to be not only meaningful, but also realistic. For example, you may need to decide on whether you can, or need to, carry out a major evaluation on several occasions. Although Laura wanted to evaluate the effectiveness of her new idea as well as whether it was happening, she did not think that she could, or needed to, repeatedly evaluate its effectiveness. She planned the initial evaluation after the first week to capture whether or not the new paperwork was used. However, at this point she did not consider it feasible to evaluate its effectiveness, because there would not have been time for this to be demonstrated. So, she carried out an audit of the charts of all the patients who were admitted that week, to see if the new assessment forms had been completed, the appropriate care plan entries made, and the stickers used. In the second evaluation, a month after implementation, she not only repeated this process but also spoke to patients and their relatives to see what their experiences of mealtime assistance had been, and discussed with staff the pros and cons of the new way of working. By doing this, she aimed to establish not only whether the mealtime initiative was happening, but also whether it was practical for staff to use, and having a positive effect for patients. At the six-month and one-year evaluations, she did not repeat the discussions with staff and patients, because the benefits or downsides of this way of working had already been explored, and were unlikely to change. At this stage, she felt she simply needed to know if the new way of working was still functioning.

Although interviews or discussions with staff and families were only carried out once, Laura had other less formal opportunities to evaluate the mealtime initiative. She paid attention to whether any complaints or compliments about the new system were made, and included these in the evaluations. This not only gave her information that was important in assessing the implementation of the project, but reminded people that, even when a formal evaluation was not taking place, she was aware of what was happening in relation to the new way of working.

Ongoing evaluation, accompanied by feedback, can help to sustain people's focus on, and interest in, a new way of working.

Planning Ongoing Developments

It has been suggested that change is more likely to be sustained if it is part of a cycle of events in which evaluation heralds further refinement and development rather than being a linear event that ends with evaluation (Parkin 2009: 110). Continually evaluating, tweaking and refining an innovation makes it very difficult to go back to square one, because the change has become a part of something bigger, and square one no longer exists. To this end, as well as monitoring and feeding back on the progress of the new system, Laura looked at ways in which she and her team could further develop the work they had begun. One idea was to have mealtime volunteers who could easily be directed to patients who needed assistance simply by using the existing sticker system. Another option that was suggested was to develop the original innovation by it being more widely used within the hospital.

Laura found that after six months the project seemed to be going well, and had positive reviews. She therefore asked her manager if any other wards were interested in using it. Although it can be easy to assume that other people know what you are doing, they often do not (Morrow et al. 2010). It turned out that the ward opposite Laura's, which was also an orthopaedic ward, did not really know what had been done on her ward: they only knew that they had a system aimed at improving things at mealtimes. When Laura met their ward manager, he thought that his ward should also trial it. Once the system was being used on both wards, there was less chance of omissions to documentation about mealtime support when staff were moved across wards, staff from both wards knew what the green stickers indicated, and some practicalities such as ordering supplies of stickers were easier because both wards used them. The green sticker status on the dependency forms also became more established as another ward took it on. This made the initiative harder to ignore, abandon, or casually neglect.

In addition to the benefits of sustaining change, this type of ongoing development from an original change has links with the concept of emancipatory practice development, where one development in practice heralds further developments, and individuals and processes as well as discrete events are developed (Wilson and McCormack 2006). Although the ward staff had not all bought into this change at the outset, it was a practitioner-led innovation, in response to a practice-based need, and had been seen to have a positive effect on care provision. It had given Laura and those who worked closely with her confidence that they had the skills and ability to change practice, and to create ongoing developments from this. In terms of emancipatory practice development, this meant that whilst a particular aspect of care was improved, individuals were also developed (Hall and Hord 2011: 2). Whilst Laura's original intention had only been to improve mealtime assistance, the outcome of her activities was that, as well as the innovation itself, she developed a new outlook on how she could initiate innovations in practice. She also began to develop her skills in reflecting critically on the way things were done, and her own and her colleagues' values, priorities, and ways of working. By doing so, she began to move her practice development activities towards a transformational approach, in which the way she thought about her work was challenged and changed. Having the opportunity to lead and succeed in managing a change in practice, Laura and those working with her were able to begin to move towards developing a culture where critical reflection on practice, and practitioner-led innovation was nurtured (Manley and McCormack 2003, Dewing 2010, Walsh et al. 2011).

Creating further developments from an innovation make it harder for the initial change to be abandoned or eroded.

Keeping People Informed

Like all aspects of the change process, a key element of sustaining new practice is communication. Communication should use any and every channel that is appropriate: meetings, emails, newsletters, posters, whatever reaches those who are involved and those whom you want to tell. Laura fed back at ward meetings after each evaluation event, but she also used email, the communication book, and posters around the ward to update people who could not come to meetings, and to reinforce the messages given. She aimed to make it almost impossible to miss anyone out, or for people to deliberately avoid seeing the information.

Keeping everyone informed of what is happening, as well as providing an opportunity for them to respond to updates, reminds everyone of events, and indicates that their opinions and feelings still matter (Giangreco and

Peccei 2005, Hall and Hord 2011: 150–152). This can be useful in terms of picking up on opposition that could slowly erode your project, keeping those who are wavering on board, and finding out about unexpected problems or glitches. Laura made sure that her feedback included problems that had been highlighted, and how they had been addressed. She included any issues that she had heard about in informal ways as well as those identified through formal evaluations, and thus aimed to give the impression that not only was she acting on feedback, but that she was aware of what was happening on the ward day to day (Giangreco and Peccei 2005, Hall and Hord 2011: 145).

Informing people about the outcome of innovations includes letting people outside your immediate group of colleagues know what has happened, and publicising successes (Golden 2006). This is important in terms of rewarding the effort of those involved, and because it clarifies that what has happened is worthwhile. It does not necessarily stop people on your own territory slipping back into old ways, but it is one more reminder that change has happened, and is expected to continue. Laura asked her manager if the project could be highlighted in the Trust newsletter. She also had an almost permanent display about the mealtime initiative on the ward notice board, which was visible to relatives and staff. She felt that, as well as keeping the project at the forefront of people's minds, this latter measure would enable patients or their relatives to ask staff about the system if they did not see it in evidence. Involving service users in strategies to maintain new practice has been highlighted as important (Virani et al. 2009), and although this might only be a small part of sustaining the mealtime initiative, Laura considered it to be a potentially important addition to the impetus.

Ongoing communication about an innovation, and the continued progress made from it, stops it from disappearing from sight as other projects come along.

Summary

Once new practice has been established, with apparent success, there is still a need to work on maintaining it. There is always a risk of people slipping back into old ways, either unintentionally or by those who oppose change persuading them to revert to previous ways of working. It can be useful to avoid claiming success to early on in the process of change, and instead to celebrate the roll out of new practice, whilst emphasising that the initiative, and effort required for it, is ongoing. This can be aided by continuing evaluation and feedback, planning ongoing practice development from the initial project, keeping people informed of developments, and sharing evidence of the success of the new way of working.

Key Points

Planning change should include how new practice will be maintained after the initial implementation.

Continued evaluation and feedback can help to sustain enthusiasm for change.

Planning ongoing practice development may make it harder for innovations to be eroded. Disseminating information about a new way of working can sustain motivation for change.

CASE STUDY

Antoniana and four other staff have been involved in introducing a new way of working with the family (or significant others) of patients who are discharged from the acute psychiatric inpatient service where they work. The initiative was developed because of an apparent increase in the number of patients who were readmitted shortly after discharge because of a lack support from their families, a perceived lack of awareness by families of what the person's needs were or who was expected to meet them, or a lack of confidence in how best to support them. The initiative involves patients and families who want to use this approach meeting with staff several times prior to the patient's discharge to discuss and confirm: what their needs are, how their needs will be met, what agreed plans of action exist, the best way to manage situations that may arise, and where to go for help or additional support.

Not everyone was in favour of the initiative. The time that it would take, concerns over whether relatives or significant others should be involved in this way, doubts over its efficacy, and a feeling that this was currently done informally anyway, were the key reasons for opposing its introduction. However, the new way of working was rolled out for patients who wished to use it. Evaluations from staff, patients and relatives were positive, and the rate of readmissions seemed to reduce. The next task was to maintain this way of working.

Were There Any Individuals or Groups Who Never Supported the Change?

Some staff did not support this initiative. The reasons that were given were that families would generally not want to attend meetings to plan discharge, that there were potential problems over confidentiality of information, and clarity of responsibility, if relatives were involved, and that it would be difficult to organise and facilitate meetings because of work schedules. Those who opposed the idea were also not convinced it would have any effect on readmission rates because they felt that this type of information was already informally shared with families where appropriate.

Although there was a small core group of staff who were enthusiastic about the new way of working, there was also a large majority who, whilst being quite happy for the innovation to go ahead, were not particularly concerned about whether it happened or not. Antoniana knew that this majority could easily be won over by those who opposed the new way of working.

Would Other Priorities Develop over Time?

There were soon other priorities, which competed with Antoniana's initiative for staff time and interest. She and her team sought to maintain the momentum for their innovation by including whether the meetings were offered or not on the standard discharge preparation documentation to remind people about them. They also gave monthly updates on what was happening, and initially congratulated people on the successful roll out, but emphasised that the project still required support and input from everyone. As time went on, they continued to give feedback about progress, what was going well, any difficulties that were encountered, how these were resolved, and the apparent outcomes of the service. Where they presented evaluation data, they compared this with how things were pre-project, and reminded people of why the initiative had been launched. This last point was intended to stop people from forgetting that the new way of working had been developed in response to a problem, not because of a personal whim or unsolicited idea from those involved in developing it.

Was There a Potential for People to Think that no Further Effort Was Required?

Although Antoniana and her team gave feedback to their colleagues a month after the new initiative was rolled out, thanked everyone for their efforts, and stated that things were going well, they emphasised that this was just the beginning. They gave information on what was being tweaked, what needed more attention, and generally aimed to give the impression that whilst they were pleased with the initiative and everyone's contribution, there was still effort required and that they were continuing to monitor events. They continued to check whether patients had been offered the chance to have pre-discharge meetings. On occasions when they discovered that this had not happened, they documented in the patient's notes that they had now offered this, the outcome, and mentioned it to the person managing that patient's care. The intention of this was not only to ensure that what they had done was communicated, but also to give the message that they were continuing to note what was happening, and not relaxing their efforts.

Were the Necessary Resources Available in the Long Term?

The main resource needed for this initiative was staff time, which had to be found from within the existing staffing resource. The time required to arrange and hold meetings was therefore an issue from the outset. However, by working with people and encouraging them to plan when meetings would happen, keeping these as a priority, and feeding back the positive results of the initiative, Antoniana and her team aimed to encourage people to see, and continue to see, this as a valid use of their time.

Was Continuing Education and Training Available?

The staff on the unit were all given input into the intention, and proposed content, of discussions with relatives. Antoniana and her team also offered opportunities for staff to discuss how particular sessions went, debrief on any difficulties or uncertainties, and share successes. They added input on pre-discharge discussions with patients and relatives to new staff induction packages, to ensure that all the staff who worked on the unit continued to be aware of this part of discharge planning.

Could Any Losses for Individuals or Groups Develop over Time?

Because there had been no formal input for relatives before this initiative, there was not felt to be likely to be any particular losses as a result of the change in practice. However, one of the staff who opposed this approach had been involved in the initial design of the current discharge plan ten years previously. She might have felt that the introduction of an addition to her work in some way undermined it. As she was opposed to the new way of working and seemed to expect it to fail, she might feel ongoing loss as the initiative took shape and showed success. This might mean that her opposition increased, rather than reduced, over time. Antoniana and her team had always stressed that their project did not change the existing discharge planning, but was meant to be used as an adjunct to it. They continued to emphasise this as the innovation became established.

Did Any Promised Benefits Materialise?

The key benefits that it had been suggested might arise from the new way of working were that if families were better prepared to support patients on discharge, readmissions would potentially reduce, or families of readmitted patients would have more established working relationships with the inpatient services. In the evaluation of the new system, and providing feedback on this, the focus was not just on whether the meetings were happening, but their effectiveness, for example, whether less patients were readmitted, what the problems that required readmission were, a comparison of readmission rates for patients who had and had not been involved in pre-discharge meetings, and how relatives contributed to discussions with staff on readmission. Wherever possible, as well as statistical information, Antoniana illustrated her feedback with examples of things that had gone well, or cited examples of relatives' positive interactions with staff, so that people could link the initiative to real experiences. She also contrasted previous statistics and experiences with those now encountered, to remind everyone of the improvements that had been made.

Was There Any Ongoing Evaluation?

The initial evaluation one month after the introduction of the new system only showed whether or not discharge meetings were happening. Although readmissions were also commented on, and appeared to have improved, it was too early to have any really meaningful data on this. After two months, a second evaluation not only showed whether the meetings were happening, but also included readmission data and interviews with staff, patients, and relatives who had used the system. The intention of this was to show not only whether the system was still being used, but it's pros, cons, and effectiveness from the point of view of all those affected by it.

A further evaluation of the system was carried out at six months, and a final evaluation at one year after implementation. These evaluations were only intended to show if the system was still being used, readmission rates, and to enable any variations in use over time, or at particular points in the year, to be seen.

Were There Further Developments from the Initial Project?

The initial initiative appeared to be working well six months after being rolled out, so Antoniana and her team considered how to develop it. One suggestion was to introduce the idea of relatives being involved in weekly meetings during the patients' hospitalisation, so that the discharge meetings became a natural continuation of this. Another idea was to introduce this initiative on other acute wards.

Were People Kept Informed of What Was Happening?

Initially, the progress of the project was reported on at each ward meeting, in the communication book, and the ward staff email newsletter. These reports diminished over time, but when formal evaluations were conducted, this was fed into meetings and emails, and noted in the communication book. Any particularly good feedback was fed into the staff communication systems at once, as were any problems that occurred, alongside how these were resolved. The intention of these unplanned reports was to remind everyone that the initiative was still in progress, and that the team were aware of, and monitoring, events. It also showed that any problems or challenges would be taken seriously and acted on, but the initiative would not be abandoned without good reason.

The initiative was reported on at liaison group meetings, and multidisciplinary team meetings, so that it was highlighted at every opportunity. The intention was not only to keep people informed, and to keep the momentum for change, but to indicate to those who opposed the project that it was becoming established, and generally seen as a core part of the support offered to patients.

GUIDED WORK

This section revisits the learning outcomes covered in the chapter. You may want to complete it alone, or with colleagues.

1. Identify factors that will assist in sustaining change.

Identify a change in practice that initially succeeded. Consider what may have contributed to it being, or not being, sustained after its initial success. You might include:

*   Whether there were any individuals or groups who never supported the change, and how their opposition was addressed.
*   Whether other priorities developed over time, and how this affected the innovation.
*   Whether people might have thought that no further effort was required and how this was managed.
*   Whether the necessary resources were available long term.
*   Whether continuing education/training needs were in place.
*   Whether losses that might accrue over time were considered.
*   Whether any promised benefits materialised.

- Whether people were kept informed of what was happening over time.
- Whether there were any further developments from or of the new way of working.

2. Appreciate the significance of continued post-innovation evaluation and feedback in sustaining change.

For the change you identified above, outline any ongoing evaluation and feedback that was carried out (if you were not directly responsible for the innovation, this may be any that you were aware of).

- For each aspect of this evaluation and feedback, consider whether this would have contributed to the innovation being sustained.
- Could any more evaluation or feedback have been usefully used?

3. Perceive the importance of continued practice developments in sustaining new ways of working.

Consider whether there were any ongoing developments associated with the innovation described above.

- If there were, did this contribute to the maintenance of the innovation?
- Would there have been any other options to develop things further?

Additional Resources

http://www.institute.nhs.uk/documents/Useful%20Templates/P_LEAD_SI_POSTERS_JAN22.pdf

http://www.institute.nhs.uk/sustainability_model/general/welcome_to_sustainability.html

http://www.clahrc-northwestlondon.nihr.ac.uk/inc/files/documents/sustainability-resources/sustainability_model_and_guide.pdf

11

Disseminating New Evidence

Chapter Learning Outcomes

After studying this chapter, the reader will be able to:

- Identify local, national, and international opportunities to share information about innovations
- Plan which aspects of an innovation might be presented at a conference
- Determine how an innovation might be presented as a journal article.

Summary

If you have been involved in developing a new way of working, you have information that is likely to be useful to other practitioners. This chapter discusses the value and practicalities of sharing innovations though local dissemination, and by means of publications and conference presentations.

Joy works on a day surgery unit where a problem arose because an increasing number of patients who had been deemed to be ready for discharge felt unable to go home. In addition, a rising number sought advice and sometimes readmission to the surgical ward on their first night post-operatively. This created difficulties for the patients concerned, the day surgery unit, and the surgical directorate as a whole. Having identified what the key issues seemed to be, Joy took the lead role in developing a new information package for patients. This included changing the information that was given to provide more realistic and specific information about what they would need to have in place at home, what they should expect, what they should or should not be concerned about, and why. This was made available not only in written format as had always been the case, but also via on a page on the hospital website. The information about what to expect was provided prior to admission, but was reissued on discharge, as the analysis of the problem showed that many patients did not have this information to hand once they got home.

The new approach to information giving was rolled out six months ago and there has been a steady decline in delayed discharge, telephone queries, and readmissions. Joy now wants to share what the unit has achieved.

Sharing Locally

Making the outcome of any change in practice known is important (Hall and Hord 2011: 154). Everyone who has given time and effort to a project should not only be told about the outcome of their work as a matter of courtesy, but also because unless they know the results of their efforts there is no reason for them to assist with ongoing or future endeavours (Pryjmachuk 1996, Skinner 2004). In addition to those who have been instrumental in implementing change, everyone who has been affected by it should know what has happened as a result of it. If people hear that a project has had positive outcomes, it may assist in gaining their ongoing co-operation, or reducing their opposition to it. Hearing what the outcome of the new way of working is, and what is happening about it now, will also serve as a reminder that the innovation is ongoing. So, when you are thinking about how to share the outcomes of a change in practice, it is worth thinking through everyone who has been involved in or affected by it, and how you can disseminate information to them.

In Joy's case, the manager of the day surgery unit had agreed to her and some colleagues having the time and resources to develop the new style of information giving, and the staff on the unit, including nursing staff, medical staff, and administration staff, had all been involved in the innovation to some extent. Staff on the general surgical wards had also been affected by the initial problems that led to the innovation, and given varying degrees of input into its development. Outside the surgical directorate, The Trust governance group had approved the process of developing a new system of giving information, the Patient Advice and Liaison Service (PALS) had helped Joy to access ex-patients to gain their views on the existing and proposed information giving system and content, and the web team had worked with her on providing information via a link on the Trust's website.

Joy not only thought about how she could feed back to individuals and groups, but also considered who should be involved in the process of feeding back. Involving the people who have been a part of developing and implementing change in publicising its outcomes can be a means of rewarding them for their efforts, keeping them on board, and developing their interest in the innovation. Joy was conscious that whilst she had led the change, she had had two key assistants on the unit. She wanted to be sure that she was not seen as taking the glory for what was a joint effort, and felt that the right thing would be for her and these two colleagues to be named in the feedback, with acknowledgments also given to the unit as a whole, colleagues on the surgical unit, the PALS service, patients who had contributed, and the web team.

Although it is natural to think that the people who are directly involved know the outcomes of changes that they are involved in, they may not (Morrow et al. 2010). Joy therefore arranged a formal means of providing feedback to the day surgery unit, via ward meetings, in the communication book, and on the staff email. She and her two key colleagues also made a poster about the new approach to discharge advice to display on the unit notice board. The poster was placed in an area where patients as well as staff could see it, which Joy hoped would be an additional reminder to them about the information they had, and what they did and did not need to be concerned about post-discharge. Joy fed back to the general surgical wards via email, their communication books, and by attending a staff meeting on each ward, so that they knew the outcome of the project, and about its ongoing implementation.

The Trust governance group required a report on how the innovation had progressed, and Joy contacted the PALS service to enquire how she could best feed back to them and the ex-patients involved. They asked her to write a short piece for their newsletter. This was useful to both parties: for PALS it highlighted an example of the value of involving patients, and how their service could influence developments in care provision. For Joy and her colleagues, it gave wider circulation to news about the project and forged a continued link with PALS. Joy wrote to the ex-patients who had participated, to let them know individually about the success of the new system of information giving, and thank them for their input. She fed back directly to the person in the web team whom she had been working with, and also felt that it would be useful for the Trust as a whole to be aware of the project. Although the innovation was specific to her unit, she thought that there might be some principles, which would be useful to other areas, and therefore asked if a short report on the project could be featured in the Trust newsletter, and on the website.

Share Information about the Outcome of Innovations . . .

With those who were involved
With those who were affected
With those who co-operated

> **Share Information about the Outcome of Innovations ...** *continued*
>
> ---
>
> With those who provided assistance
> With other areas of practice that might find the information useful

As well as sharing the new approach to discharge information within the hospital, Joy thought that there was something that student nurses could learn from this. She contacted one the lecturers at the university to ask if there would be any interest in her giving a short presentation to students to explain the way in which the day surgery unit had improved their discharge preparation, including the way the change in practice was set up, managed, and evaluated. The response was positive, and she and her colleagues presented this work in the third year developing practice unit. This gave useful input to the students, and helped Joy and her colleagues to increase their confidence in giving presentations, which was valuable when they came to consider presenting at conferences.

Sharing information about an innovation enables you to highlight your work and that of others, and to strengthen collaborations that have developed during the project.

Publicising Your Work Outside Your Workplace

As well as feeding back to those most closely involved in, or affected by, a change in practice, publicising your work outside your immediate workplace has benefits. If you have done something new, the chances are that others could learn from it and develop their practice too. You may feel that a change in practice, which you have effected, is just a small project, and not important enough to publish. However, many practitioners want or need to carry out small-scale innovations, and learning about what other individuals or teams have done can be very beneficial (Happell 2008). When she designed the new information for patients, Joy found relatively little information to help her. It would have been useful for her to have been able to read an example of how another unit had approached developing patient information, what worked, and what did not. The key issue is not so much whether your project is extensive enough to merit sharing it with others, as whether you can accurately pull out the key issues that would matter to other people who are trying a similar thing, and explain why what worked did, and why what did not work did not. If no one knows what works, what does not work, and the new ideas that are being tried out, everyone has to do all the background work time and time again.

Useful Things to Share about Your Innovation

What you have done.
Why you did it.
How you did it.
What the outcome was.
What worked well.
What didn't work.

Publicising your work also raises your profile and that of anyone else involved. Two approaches to getting information about your innovation into the public domain are publication and conference presentations. How you choose to publicise your work is partly a matter of personal preference and circumstance: if you are more confident in speaking than writing, then conference presentations may be a good place to start. If you are more confident with writing, written publications may be your best option.

Publication

There are a range of journals that you can publish in, and the first step is probably deciding who you want to tell about your work, for example, whether your message is aimed at practitioners, managers, or academics. It is also useful to think about exactly who within that broad category you want to target: if you want to target practitioners, do you mean practitioners generally, or those in a specific area? Are the practitioners from one profession, or more than one (Happell 2008, Price 2010)? Joy really wanted to let other nurses working on day surgery units know about what her unit had done, so she looked for journals aimed at practitioners. She was, however, open to the idea of writing for either a general nursing journal, or one focused specifically on surgery or day care surgery, depending on what was available and appropriate.

There are various places where you can search for the journals that exist, such as

http://en.wikipedia.org/wiki/List_of_nursing_journals,
http://www.rcn.org.uk/development/researchanddevelopment/kt/
dissemination/publish#database.

Having identified journals that might be suitable, you can visit their websites to get the information on authors, which tells you the target audience for the journal, what types of article the journal publishes, how the manuscript should be presented, and how many words an article should be. It is also a good idea to get access to at least one recent edition of the journal so that you can see if the tone and approach used in it matches what you have to present. Joy wanted to be able to write enough to give a good overview of the project, so she looked for a journal that gave at least 2500 words for articles. As she browsed the journals, she came across one nursing journal that had a section devoted to developments in practice, which could be up to 3000 words long. This seemed the best option for what she wanted to write about. She also had the option of writing for a management journal, and focusing on the change management aspect of the project. However, although she had learned some important lessons about managing change, her priority was to focus on the nursing practice aspect of the new way of giving information to patients.

Joy and her two key colleagues not only jointly authored the article, but also acknowledged other people and teams who had been instrumental in the success of the innovation. As Joy had taken the lead on the project and did most of the writing, she was named as the first author. They submitted their article to the journal of their choice, and it was returned from the reviewers asking for revisions. At first, Joy was a little crestfallen by this, because there seemed to be a lot of comments about things that she thought had been clear, and considerable extra work appeared to be required. However, after leaving it for a day and going back to it, she realised that although the comments seemed quite extensive, the work was not excessive, and would improve the article. It was mostly changing the order of things so that the flow of ideas was more logically presented, and providing additional explanations so that someone who had not been involved could understand the project better. Having gone to the effort of initially writing it, she would be wasting a lot of existing work not to make the changes. She and her colleagues revised the article, and it was subsequently accepted.

Conferences

As well as writing for publication, conferences are an option for getting your work known about more widely. There are numerous conferences, targeting different audiences, with different focuses, to select from, and several websites listing them, such as

http://sites.google.com/site/consumerconferencesevents/medical-
  conferences-2011-2012-2013-2014-listings-by-specialism/nursing-care-
  conferences-congresses-2011-2012-2013-2014-us-uk-europe-asia-world,
http://www.rcn.org.uk/newsevents/events,
http://www.conferencealerts.com/topic-listing?topic=Nursing.

Trawling through the conferences that are available and deciding what you want to present, to which audience, and whether you want a fairly local or national conference will help you to decide where to focus your efforts. Some of this again depends on your confidence, experience, personal circumstances, and preferences. Some people choose to start small at a local conference, and look at larger options later, as their confidence develops. Alternatively, if there is an international conference that is relevant, and which gives you a chance to extend your networks and go travelling to somewhere interesting, that can be a very good option too.

Joy could have chosen to present at a management-focused conference, a conference about nursing practice in general, a conference specific to surgical nursing or day surgery. She ideally wanted to keep her focus on the day surgery aspect of her work, and to address clinical rather than managerial issues. She therefore looked for conferences focused on day surgery.

Conference presentations usually give choices about the format you would like to present in: most have options for posters and oral presentations. Your choice will be affected by your preferences, but you may also have to consider funding because some organisations prefer to fund people to attend conferences if they are giving oral presentations rather than presenting posters. That is something to check locally because if all things are equal but you will be funded for one option and not the other, the choice may be obvious. Joy was not very confident about standing up to present her work to an audience, but at the same time she wanted to meet with other people and share ideas, so she and her colleagues applied to present a poster at a day surgery conference. Her unit agreed to fund their places at the conference, but could not give them additional time off to attend. Having been to the conference, and presented the poster, Joy thought that if she was involved in another project she would like to try to attend a conference to present a verbal report at a concurrent session. Her own NHS Trust was hosting a conference about innovations in care and her manager suggested that they put together a session for this as there would be no cost involved for attendance or travel. This seemed a good idea, and enabled Joy and her colleagues to gain the experience of presenting on home territory.

There is no best way to share your experiences and findings: it depends who you want to tell, what you want to say, and how you want to say it.

Letting People Know What Doesn't Work and Why

Although the aim of disseminating evidence on change is often described in terms of advertising successes, as Chapter 9 outlined, not all change projects achieve their initial aims. If the things that people have invested in do not work out as planned, they need to know about this, why this was, and what will happen next. It would have been important for Joy to give feedback to all those who had been involved or contributed to her work, even if the project had not gone to plan, so that those concerned could see why their efforts seemed not to have had the outcomes they had expected. As well as feeding back to those directly involved, it is useful to consider publishing or presenting about the process or outcomes of change projects that do not achieve their aims. There is a world of difference between publicly castigating yourself and others, and sharing why an idea did not work out in practice. If someone else is planning to do what you did and can hear whether it really will work in practice or not, and about what might have caused problems or made things go better, it can stop them from falling into known pitfalls, or embarking on a project that has no chance of success. Sharing the outcomes of change which has not met its original aim includes not only exploring whether things could have been done differently, but also highlighting any positive outcomes from it. It may seem very altruistic to advertise your struggles so that others can learn from them: but you do get a publication, or conference presentation, for all the trouble you have gone to, and it is a significant contribution to what is known about practice.

It can be just as useful for other people to hear about what did not work well as what did; otherwise, the same problems will need to be addressed again and again.

Summary

When you are planning making the outcomes of a change in practice known, you should identify who within your own immediate workplace and organisation needs to know about the outcomes, and the best and most useful way of providing this information. It is also worth considering how you can make your work known to a wider audience, through publications or conference presentations. This may include not only sharing information on change that has been successful, but also elements of change that have not gone to plan, or had the desired or expected outcomes.

Having planned, implemented, evaluated, and publicised a change in practice, you are finally entitled to a sit down with a cup of tea and cake, until you begin the next stage of or idea for practice development.

CASE STUDY

Joy and her colleagues selected and planned their poster presentation and publication as follows.

What Conference Did Joy and Her Colleagues Select?

Joy and her colleagues selected a conference focused on day surgery at which to present their poster. The focus of the conference that they selected was nursing practice in day surgery. Joy found this by searching for day surgery conferences having heard from her colleagues that they thought there was an annual day surgery nursing conference.

What Did Joy and Her Colleagues Decide to Include in the Conference Presentation?

Joy and her colleagues could present a poster up to A3 size. They started their planning with a list of the things they could present about their project. These included identifying what the problem and its cause were, deciding what could be done to address it, the process of designing the new information, how they managed the process of change, and what the outcomes of the new way of giving information were.

When they looked at the space they had, they realised that this would be too much for one poster, and that if they tried to include it all, the poster would become crowded and uninviting. They therefore decided to aim to give a summary that would draw people to discuss their project with them. This would include a statement of what the problem was found to be (rather than the process of problem analysis), how they decided to address it, how they decided what to put in the new leaflet as well as on the website, an example of the contents, and the findings from the evaluation. Each section would be brief, outlining a few key points that anyone viewing the poster could discuss with them in more detail.

They divided the poster into five areas as shown in Figure 11.1, so as to have each section of information clearly delineated from the others, for ease of reading. They also aimed to make the poster attractive by including two or three relevant photos or illustrations. When their poster was accepted, Joy checked whether there would be internet connection available at the

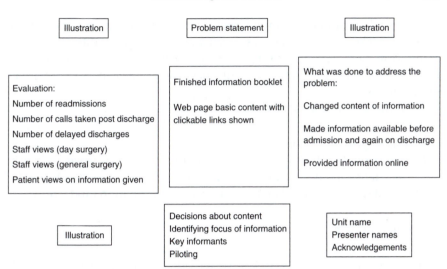

Figure 11.1 Poster outline

conference, so that they could, if requested, show people on a laptop how the web link for patient information worked.

What Journal Did Joy and Her Colleagues Select?

Joy and her colleagues searched three lists of nursing journals to find the right one to publish in. Although they had ideally wanted to find a journal focused on day surgery or surgical nursing, the one that seemed to accept articles of the type they wanted to write, and specifically invited discussions of innovations in practice, was a general nursing journal.

What Did Joy and Her Colleagues Include in Their Article?

The journal guidelines gave a word limit of 3000 words, excluding the reference list and figures. The tone of the journal was to focus on clear messages for practice, based on sound rationale, which drew not only on theory but also on experience.

Joy and her colleagues had to decide what aspect of their work they would present in the article. They decided that their main focus would be to look at what they changed in the information leaflet, why they changed things in the way they did, and to what end, as this was likely to be what was most relevant to other practitioners. By focusing on why they changed things, and the general way in which things were changed, rather than the specific details of what particular content they had in the new information, they hoped to make points which nurses outside day surgery units might find useful. However, they included figures of selected aspects of the information given to patients to illustrate the points made, and to give ideas to other day surgery units.

Their initial plan for their work was as follows:

Article length: 3000 words
Introduction: Set the scene of where the innovation happened, and why the change in approach to information giving was needed (300 words)
The limitations of the existing way of giving information (400 words)

The new design:

Involvement of patients as key stakeholders in design (reasons, challenges) (400 words)
Change in how patient expectations were managed: more realistic information (400 words)
Change in level of information given (explanation of reasons for common post-operative symptoms and why these were not a cause for concern) (350 words)
Web page with clickable links to give a range of information options (and reasons for this being used) (250 words)
Repeated provision of information leaflet (and reasons for this) (200 words)
Evaluation of the project with a focus on the outcomes rather than process of evaluation (400 words)
Summary (300 words)

The word counts they allocated to each section were movable, but at the planning stage they wanted to get some idea of whether they were allocating enough space for each issue, and equally if they were overestimating what they had to say for each part. These sections also clarified the key messages that they felt were important: namely, to give advice that was realistic, did not create false expectations, and was easily accessible, and to emphasise the value of including patients in designing the information.

As they wrote the article, the lengths and emphasis of each section changed slightly, but the initial plan had given them a good place to start working from.

GUIDED WORK

This section revisits the learning outcomes covered in the chapter. You may want to complete it alone, or with colleagues.

1. Identify local opportunities to share information about innovations.

List ways in which you have, or could share, the outcomes of a change in practice that you have been involved in with

- Your immediate colleagues.
- Your organisation as a whole.
- Other teams who collaborated with you.
- Other local organisations or teams.

2. Plan which aspects of an innovation might be presented at a conference.

In relation to a change in practice that you have been involved in:

- Look for a conference that you could present your work at.
- List the things that you would include in your conference presentation.

3. Determine how an innovation might be presented as a journal article.

In relation to a change in practice which you have been involved in:

- Look for a journal that you could publish your work in.
- Look at their guidelines for authors and plan what you would include in your article.

Additional Resources

Writing for publication:
https://www.msu.edu/~budzynda/nursing/publishing.html   and   http://www.nurseauthoreditor.com/WritingforPublication2009.pdf

Presenting at conferences:
http://www.rcn.org.uk/development/communities/rcn_forum_communities/

Additional Resources *continued*

orthopaedic_and_trauma/news_stories/inspiration,_passion_and_commitment_
a_conference_experience www.rcn.org.uk/__data/assets/word_doc/0010/59824/
poster.doc   http://nurse-practitioners-and-physician-assistants.advanceweb.com/
Archives/Article-Archives/Presenting-at-conferences-Rewarding-start-to-finish.
aspx

Endpoints

One of the few certainties in life is that things will change. However, when change involves people altering the way they work, it can be difficult to bring about, and even more difficult to maintain. Because of this, if you are involved in introducing a change in practice, thinking about why and how you will achieve this merits as much thought as deciding what it is that you intend should be done differently.

Planning an innovation in practice includes deciding whether the change you want to make primarily involves people doing something particular, and possibly procedural, in a new way, or whether you intend to use a particular change in practice as a platform to work with people on developing an approach to their work that incorporates the ethos of ongoing practice development. This will influence how the change is planned, the way in which people are involved in it, and whether the initiative is seen as a one-off event, or as a part of a larger practice development process.

Deciding what needs to change, and why, is an important first step in planning any proposed change in practice. This includes thinking about whether a new way of working is needed because a problem has been identified, which requires a resolution; because of a new policy, protocol, or strategy being introduced; or because there is evidence that something could possibly be done in a different way and seems worth trying. Being clear about why a change in practice is being proposed means that you can explain the reason for change to those who will need to be involved in, or are likely to be affected by, it and consider how this may influence whether or not people will be enthusiastic about changing the way they work.

Once the general principles of what needs to change and why have been decided on, it is useful to develop clear aims and objectives from this, to further clarify exactly what needs to change, and to what end. This helps you to be sure that what you plan to do does address or relate to the original reason for proposing change. It also means that you can see exactly what you need to achieve, and thus what actions you will need to take and what will need to be put in place to enable this to happen.

Having decided what your aims and objectives are, you have a direction from which to begin to plan the detail of how you will manage the process of change. Although the practicalities of this, such as the resources needed, and timing and sequence of events are important, equally, and often even more important, is thinking about how you will recruit and retain enough support for your project. A key aspect of planning change is thinking about how to improve the support and enthusiasm your project attracts from your peers and mangers. Strategies to increase the support that you have can include involving people in designing the new way of working, and planning change in a way that creates as good as possible a fit between it and other organisational and personal priorities. It is also useful to consider how the proposed change may affect individuals and groups, what it will mean for them, and why people might or might not welcome it. This analysis of the things, which may help or hinder your efforts to change practice, includes thinking about specific aspects of your innovation that may create resistance to it, including individual and corporate experiences of change, other concurrent or recent changes, the basis of the evidence of a need for change, the effects that change may have on individual circumstances and lifestyles, change creating feelings of loss, and fear or apprehension about a new way of working. Thinking about the things that are likely to influence the acceptance or otherwise of change should mean that you have a good idea of whether, in terms of human and material resources, there is enough force supporting or driving change to overcome any resistance or forces that may restrain change. This enables you to make a judgment as to whether the individuals and team concerned are ready enough for change to go ahead, or whether more work has to be done before an innovation can be developed further.

When you are planning change, it is also important to consider who the key players will be, who the opinion leaders are, and how their responses to change will affect the responses of others. These may be people who are obviously influential, such as managers, or people with formal roles related to the proposed change. Equally though, they may be individuals who have no obvious reason to influence change, but whose opinions count and who are respected and listened to. A key aspect of planning change is considering how key players and opinion leaders can be brought on board and used to positively influence change, and, if they cannot, how you can manage their indifference or opposition.

A further decision about how to bring about change is to decide how it might best be implemented. This includes whether to gradually phase in a new way of working, carry out an initial pilot followed by wider adoption if the pilot is successful, or to use a one-off, 'big bang' method of implementing a new way of working. The decision as to which approach is best will be influenced not only by the reasons for change being proposed or required, but also by the assessments you have made about the forces that are likely to drive or restrain change, and how these will be affected by the chosen approach to implementing new practice. Many changes in healthcare will affect more than one discipline. The stages and considerations involved in planning and rolling out change, therefore, often have to take into account groups and individuals from within and across disciplines, and how they will affect and be affected by a new way of working.

Once the planning and preparation is complete and change is rolled out, the next challenge is to maintain everyone's motivation, build on the support that you have, and generate more. At this point, as well as feeding back on success and highlighting positive outcomes, it is important how you manage problems, difficult situations, or setbacks. Managing difficulties effectively whilst also keeping the project on track shows that you are interested in the individuals involved, are ready to listen to their views and concerns, adapt what you can to improve things, but that you are also committed to the project, and to making it work. Recalling your initial aims and objectives is valuable at this stage, because it enables you to see what concessions or changes you can make, whilst still staying true to the core aim of the project.

Having introduced a new way of working, evaluating it is important, in order to assess whether change has really happened, its effect, and the reason for its success or otherwise. The evaluation of change should enable you to decide what needs to be done next, in order to maintain and develop the new way of working if is having a positive effect, how to adjust it to improve things further, or, if things are not working well, whether to abandon it. Not all change will go to plan, or achieve its expected outcomes; and recognising this, and deciding what to do about an innovation, which has not worked out as intended, is as important as planning what to do about successful change.

If a new way of working is having a positive effect, having implemented it, managing its maintenance is vital. There is a very real risk of individuals and groups, either inadvertently or deliberately, slipping back into old ways after change has apparently taken place, and of those who oppose a project persuading others to return to previous ways of working. Planning how to maintain successful change includes thinking about how enthusiasm for and commitment to the new way of working can be sustained. Ways of achieving this include ongoing evaluation and feedback, carrying out continued practice development initiatives from the initial project, keeping people informed of developments, showcasing success, and disseminating new evidence derived from the change in practice. Sharing the project outcomes not only locally but also nationally and internationally, for example, through conferences and publications, can be a part of this.

It has been suggested that the best way to sustain change is to develop an initial project into a cycle of continuous practice development, in which an initial innovation is developed, refined, and built upon. This reduces the possibility of the benefits of change being lost, because constant evolution means that it would be almost impossible to identify and return to a set point in the past. The more that has to be undone to return to baseline, the less likely this is to happen. From such an approach to innovation, a culture in which the development of practice, with practitioners constantly questioning what might realistically be done to improve their knowledge and the way they work, and reflecting on and questioning their approach to care provision may also be created and nurtured. In the initial stages of such cultures developing, involving others in thinking about current practice, and identifying what could change, why, and how, and in evaluating new ways of working can create a feeling of ownership of the particular change. It can also nurture a belief in the value of developing new ideas and practices, and confidence that individuals can achieve this.

In the longer term, as well as the intrinsic benefits of contributing to the development of a culture of practice development, enabling your colleagues to develop skills and confidence in instigating change means that you can occasionally step back, enjoy other aspects of life, and let someone else take on the key responsibilities involved in managing change.

Bibliography

Albrecht S. (2010) 'Understanding employee cynicism toward change in healthcare contexts', *International Journal of Information Systems and Change Management* 4, 3, 194–209.

Aleem IS, Jalal H, Aleem IS, Sheikh AA, Bhandari M. (2009) 'Clinical decision analysis: Incorporating the evidence with patient preferences', *Patient Preference and Adherence* 3, 21–24.

Allan E. (2007) 'Change management for school nurses in Scotland', *Nursing Standard* 21, 42, 35–39.

Allen I. (2000) 'Modernising the NHS. Challenges to the health services: The professions', *British Medical Journal* 320, 1533–1535.

Anderson S. (2002) 'Managing change: Theory and evidence', *Journal of Clinical Excellence* 4, 3, 339–341.

Anderson B, Klein E, Stuart J. (2000) 'Why change is a conscious choice', *The Journal for Quality and Participation*, Jan–Feb, 32–36.

Astin F. (2009) 'A beginner's guide to appraising a qualitative research paper', *British Journal of Cardiac Nursing* 4, 11, 530–533.

Atwal A, Caldwell K. (2005) 'Do all health and social care professionals interact equally: A study of interactions in multidisciplinary teams in the United Kingdom', *Scandanavian Journal of Caring Science* 19, 268–273.

Atwal A, Jones M. (2007) 'The importance of the multidisciplinary team', *British Journal of Healthcare Assistants* 19, 9, 425–428.

Austin J, Currie B. (2003) 'Changing organizations for a knowledge economy: The theory and practice of change management', *Journal of Facilities Management* 2, 3, 229–243.

Balasubramanian BA, Chase SM, Nutting PA, Cohen DJ, Strickland PA, Crosson JC, Miller WL, Crabtree BF. (2010) 'Using Learning Teams for Reflective Adaptation (ULTRA): Insights from a team-based change management strategy in primary care', *Annals of Family Medicine* 8, 5, 425–432.

Balls P. (2009) 'Phenomenology in nursing research: Methodology, interviewing and transcribing', *Nursing Times* 105, 32–33, 30–33.

Beauchamp TL, Childress JF. (2001) *Principles of Biomedical Ethics* (Oxford, Oxford University Press).

Bennett M. (2003) 'Implementing new clinical guidelines: The manager as agent of change', *Nursing Management* 10, 7, 20–23.

Bigelow B, Arndt M. (2005) 'Transformational change in health care: Changing the question', *Hospital Topics* 83, 2, 19–26.

Blamey A, Mackenzie M. (2007) 'Theories of change and realistic evaluation: Peas in a pod or apples and oranges?', *Evaluation* 13, 4, 439–455.

Burck C. (2005) 'Comparing qualitative research methodologies for systemic research: The use of grounded theory, discourse analysis and narrative analysis', *Journal of Family Therapy* 27, 3, 237–262.

Burla L, Knierim B, Barth J, Liewad K, Duetz M, Abel T. (2008) 'From text to codings', *Nursing Research* 57, 2, 113–117.

Burton C. (2004) *Understanding How Research Is Presented* (London, Distance Learning Centre, South Bank University).

Cameron E, Green M. (2009) *Making Sense of Change Management: A Complete Guide to the Models, Tools and Techniques of Organizational Change*, 2nd edn (London, Kogan Page).

Campos CJG, Turato ER. (2009) 'Content analysis in studies using the clinical-qualitative method: Application and perspectives', *Revista Latino-Americana de Enfermagem* 17, 2, 259–264.

Carr A. (2000) 'Critical theory and the psychodynamics of change: A note about organizations as therapeutic settings', *Journal of Organizational Change Management* 13, 3, 289–299.

Carroll J, Quijada M. (2004) 'Redirecting traditional professional values to support safety: Changing organizational culture in healthcare', *Quality and Safety in Healthcare* 13 supplement ii, 16–21.

Chin R, Benne KD. (1985) 'General strategies for effecting change in human systems'. In Bennis WD, Benne KD, Chin R. (eds) *The Planning of Change*, 4th edn (New York, Holt Rinehart and Winston).

Choi BCK, Pak AWP. (2006) 'Multidisciplinarity, interdisciplinarity and transdisciplinarity in health research, services, education and policy: 1. Definitions, objectives, and evidence of effectiveness', *Clinical and Investigative Medicine* 29, 6, 351–364.

Clarke G. (2001) *Action Planning. Hemophilia Organization Development Monograph Series No. 2* (Montreal, Quebec, Canada, World Federation of Hemophilia).

Coghlan D, McAuliffe E. (2003) *Changing Healthcare Organizations* (Dublin, Blackhall Publishing).

Comfort H. (2010) *Practical Guide to Outcome Evaluation* (London, Jessica Kingsley).

Cork A. (2005) 'A model for successful change management', *Nursing Standard* 19, 25, 40–42.

Coughlan M, Cronin P, Ryan F. (2007) 'Step by-step guide to critiquing research. Part 1. Quantitative research', *British Journal of Nursing* 16, 11, 658–663.

Creswell JW. (2003) *Research Design: Qualitative, Quantitative, and Mixed Methods Approaches*, 2nd edn (Thousand Oaks CA, Sage Publications).

Curry LA, Nembhard IM, Bradley EH. (2009) 'Qualitative and mixed methods provide unique contributions to outcomes research', *Circulation* 119, 10, 1442–1452.

Davies B, Larson J, Contro N, Reyes-Hailey C, Ablin AR, Chesla CA, Sourkes B, Cohen H. (2009) 'Conducting a qualitative culture study of pediatric palliative care', *Qualitative Health Research* 19, 1, 5–16.

de Jager P. (2001) 'Resistance to change: A new view of an old problem', *The Futurist* 35, 3, 24–27.

Dewing J. (2010) 'Moments of movement: Active learning and practice development', *Nurse Education in Practice* 10, 1, 22–26.

Doran GT. (1981) 'There's a SMART way to write management's goals and objectives', *Management Review* 70, 11, 35–36.

Eccles M, Grimashaw J, Campbell M, Ramsay C. (2003) 'Research designs for studies evaluating the effectiveness of change and improvement strategies', *Quality and Safety in Healthcare* 12, 47–52.

Erwin DG, Garman AN. (2010) 'Resistance to organizational change: Linking research and practice', *Leadership and Organizational Development Journal* 31, 1, 39–56.

European Commission. (2004) *Aid Delivery Methods. Volume 1: Project Cycle Management Guidelines* (Brussels, European Commission, Europaid Corporation Office).

Ferrance E. (2000) *Action Research* (Providence RI, Brown University).

Fitzgerald L, Ferlie E, Addicott R, Baezamsc J, Buchananba D, McGivern G. (2007) 'Service improvement in healthcare: Understanding change capacity and change context', *Clinician in Management* 15, 2, 61–74.

Fossey E, Harvey C, McDermott F, Davidson L. (2002) 'Understanding and evaluating qualitative research', *Australian and New Zealand Journal of Psychiatry* 36, 6, 717–732.

Fronda Y, Moriceau JL. (2008) 'I am not your hero: Change management and culture shocks in a public sector corporation', *Journal of Organizational Change Management* 21, 5, 589–609.

Fui-Hoon Nah F, Lee-Shang Lau J, Kuang J. (2001) 'Critical factors for successful implementation of enterprise systems', *Business Process Management Journal* 7, 3, 285–296.

Garavaglia B. (2008) 'The problem with root cause analysis', *Nursing Homes* February, 38–39.

Garbarino S, Holland J. (2009) *Quantitative and Qualitative Methods in Impact Evaluation and Measuring Results* (London, Governance and Social Development Resource Centre and Department for International Development).

Giangreco A, Peccei R. (2005) 'The nature and antecedents to middle manager resistance to change; evidence from an Italian context', *International Journal of Human Resource Management* 16, 10, 1812–1829.

Glasziou P, Vandenbroucke J, Chalmers P. (2004) 'Assessing the quality of research', *British Medical Journal* 328, 7430, 39–41.

Glenaffric Ltd. (2007) *Six Steps to Effective Evaluation: A Handbook for Programme and Project Managers* (San Francisco, Glenaffric Ltd).

Golden B. (2006) 'Change: Transforming healthcare organizations', *Healthcare Quarterly* 10 special issue, 10–19.

Goodman B. (2008) 'Crunch the numbers', *Nursing Standard* 22, 29, 49.

Gopikrishna V. (2010) 'A report on case reports', *Journal of Conservative Dentistry* 13, 4, 265–271.

Graneheim UH, Lundman B. (2004) 'Qualitative content analysis in nursing research: Concepts, procedures and measures to achieve trustworthiness', *Nurse Education Today* 24, 2, 105–112.

Grol R, Grimashaw J. (2003) 'From best evidence to best practice: Effective implementation of change in a patients' care', *The Lancet* 362, 9391, 1225–1230.

Guy K, Gibbons C. (2003) 'Doing it by yourself', *Nursing Management* 10, 6, 19–23.

Hagedorn H, Hogan M, Smith JL, Bowman C, Curran GM, Espades D, Kimmel B, Kochevar L, Legro MW, Sales AE. (2006) 'Lessons learned about implementing research evidence into clinical practice', *Journal of General Internal Medicine* 21, S21–S24.

Hahn DL. (2009) 'Importance of evidence grading for guideline implementation: The example of Asthma', *Annals of Family Medicine* 7, 4, 364–369.

Hall GE, Hord SM. (2011) *Implementing Change: Patterns, Principles and Potholes*, 3rd edn (London, Pearson).

Happell B. (2008) 'Writing for publication: A practical guide', *Nursing Standard* 22, 28, 35–40.

Harvey G, Wensing M. (2003) 'Methods for evaluation of small scale quality improvement projects', *Quality and Safety in Healthcare* 12, 210–214.

Haveri A. (2008) 'Evaluation of change in local governance: The rhetorical wall and the politics of images', *Evaluation* 14, 2, 141–155.

Hendy J, Barlow J. (2011) 'The role of the organizational champion in achieving health system change', *Social Science and Medicine* 74, 348–355.

Hewitt-Taylor J. (2011) *Using Research in Practice* (Basingstoke, Palgrave McMillan).

Higgs M, Rowland D. (2005) 'All changes great and small: Exploring approaches to change and its leadership', *Journal of Change Management* 5, 2, 121–151.

Hodges B. (2008) 'Change management: Setting up an asthma camp for children', *Nursing Standard* 23, 15–17, 35–38.

Holt DT, Armenakis AA, Harris SG, Field HS. (2007) 'Toward a comprehensive definition of readiness for change: A review of research and instrumentation', *Research in Organizational Change and Development* 16, 289–336.

Hovland. (2005) *Successful Communication, A Toolkit for Researchers and Civil Society Organizations* (London, Overseas Development Institute) http://www.odi.org.uk/resources/docs/192.pdf.

Hughes R. (2008) 'Understanding audit: Methods and application', *Nursing and Residential Care* 11, 2, 88–91.

Iles V, Cranfield S. (2004) *Managing Change in the NHS. Developing Change Management Skills: A Resource for Health Care Professionals and Managers* (London, National Co-ordinating Centre for NHS Service Delivery and Organization Research and Development).

Iles V, Sutherland K. (2001) *Organizational Change: A Review for Health Care Managers, Professionals and Researchers* (London, National Co-ordinating Centre for NHS Service Delivery and Organization Research and Development).

International Council of Nurses. (2009) *Delivering Quality, Serving Communities Nurses Leading Caring Innovations* (Geneva, International Council of Nurses).

Jimmieson NL, Peach M, White KM. (2008) 'Utilizing the theory of planned behaviour to inform change management: An investigation of employee intentions to support organizational change', *The Journal of Applied Behavioural Science* 44, 2, 237–262.

Kearney MH. (2005) 'Seeking the sound bite: Reading and writing clinically useful qualitative research', *Journal of Obstetric, Gynecologic and Neonatal Nursing* 34, 4, 417.

Kegan R, Lahey LL. (2001) 'The real reason people won't change', *Harvard Business Review* November, 85–92.

Koch T. (2006) 'Establishing rigour in qualitative research: The decision trail', *Journal of Advanced Nursing* 53, 1, 91–100.

Korner M. (2010) 'Interprofessional teamwork in medical rehabilitation: A comparison of multidisciplinary and interdisciplinary team approach', *Clinical Rehabilitation* 24, 8, 745–755.

Kotter JP. (1995) 'Leading change: Why transformation efforts fail', *Harvard Business Review* March–April, 1–10.

Krueger G. (2006) 'Meaning making in the aftermath of sudden infant death syndrome', *Nursing Inquiry* 13, 3,163–171.

Kübler Ross E. (1997) *On Death and Dying* (New York, Touchstone).

Kyriakidou O. (2011) 'Relational perspectives on the construction of meaning: A network model of change interpretation', *Journal of Organizational Change Management* 24, 5, 572–592.

Latino RJ. (2004) 'Optimizing FMEA and RCA efforts in health care', *Journal of Healthcare Risk Management* 24, 3, 21–28.

Lee P. (2006) 'Understanding and critiquing quantitative research papers', *Nursing Times* 102, 28, 28–30.

Lewin K. (1951) *Field Theory in Social Science Selected Theoretical Papers* (New York, Harper and Row).

Lincoln YS, Guba EG. (1985) *Naturalistic Inquiry* (Newbury Park, CA, Sage Publications).

LoBindo-Wood G, Haber J. (2005) *Nursing Research Methods and Critical Appraisal for Evidence Based Practice*, 6th edn (St Louis Missouri, MA, Mosby Elsevier).

Ludwick DA, Doucette J. (2009) 'The implementation of operational processes for the Alberta Electronic Health Record: Lessons from electronic medical record adoption in primary care', *Electronic Healthcare* 7, 4, 103–107.

MacPhee M, Suryaprakash N. (2012) 'First-line nurse leaders health care change management initiatives', *Journal of Nursing Management* 20, 249–259.

Manley K, McCormack B. (2003) 'Practice development: Purpose, methodology, facilitation and evaluation', *Nursing in Critical Care* 8, 1, 22–29.

McCabe D. (2010) 'Taking the long view: A cultural analysis of memory as resisting and facilitating organizational change', *Journal of Organizational Change Management* 23, 3, 230–250.

McDonnell A, Wilson R, Goodacre S. (2006) 'Evaluating and implementing new services', *British Medical Journal* 332, 109–112.

McGrath JE, Johnson BA. (2003) 'Methodology makes meaning: How both qualitative and quantitative paradigms shape evidence and its interpretation', Chapter 3, 31–38. In Camic PM, Rhodes JE, Yardley L. (eds) *Qualitative Research in Psychology: Expanding Perspectives in Methodology and Design* (Washington DC, APA Books).

McLean C. (2011) 'Change and transition: What is the difference?', *British Journal of School Nursing* 6, 2, 78–81.

McMurray A, Chaboyer W, Wallis M, Fetherston C. (2010) 'Implementing bedside handover: Strategies for change management', *Journal of Clinical Nursing* 19, 17–19, 2580–2589.

Mertens DM. (2005) *Research and Evaluation in Education and Psychology: Integrating Diversity with Quantitative, Qualitative and Mixed-methods*, 2nd edn (Thousand Oaks CA, Sage Publications).

Moon MY. (2009) 'Making sense of common sense for change management buy-in', *Management Decisions* 47, 3, 518–532.

Moran JW, Brightman BK. (1998) 'Effective management of healthcare change', *The TQM Magazine* 10, 1, 27–29.

Morrow E, Morrow E, Robert G, Maben J, Griffiths P. (2010) 'Improving healthcare quality at scale and pace. Lessons from The Productive Ward: Releasing time to care', www.institute.nhs.uk/productive ward.

Motulsky H. (1995) *Intuitive Biostatistics* (Oxford, Oxford University Press).

National Institute for Health and Clinical Excellence (NICE). (2005) 'Assessing evidence and recommendations in NICE guidelines – paper for SMT', www.nice.org.uk/niceMedia/pdf/smt/251005item3.pdf, accessed 9 September 2010.

National Institute for Health and Clinical Excellence (NICE). (2007) *How to Change Practice* (London, NICE).

National Patient Safety Agency and National Research Ethics Service. (2009) *Defining Research* (London, National Patient Safety Agency and National Research Ethics Service).

Oakland JS, Tanner SJ. (2007) 'A New Framework for managing change', *The TQM Magazine* 19, 6, 572–589.

Okes D. (2008) 'The human side of root cause analysis', *Journal for Quality and Participation* 31, 3, 20–29.

O'Neill M, Cowman S. (2007) 'Partners in care: Investigating community nurses' understanding of an interdisciplinary team-based approach to primary care', *Journal of Clinical Nursing* 17, 3004–3011.

Oreg S. (2006) 'Personality, context and resistance to organizational change', *European Journal of Work and Organizational Psychology* 15, 1, 73–101.

Oxman AD, Flottorp S. (2001) 'An overview of strategies to promote implementation of evidence-based health care', Chapter 8, 101–119. In Silagy C, Haines A. (eds) *Evidence-Based Practice in Primary Care*, 2nd edn (London, BMJ Books).

Palmer B. (2004) 'Overcoming resistance to change', *Quality Progress* 37, 4, 35–39

Parahoo K. (2006) *Nursing Research: Principles, Process and Issues*, 2nd edn (Basingstoke, Palgrave Macmillan).

Paré G, Sicotte C, Poba-Nzaou P, Balouzakis G. (2011) 'Clinicians' perceptions of organizational readiness for change in the context of clinical information system projects: Insights from two cross-sectional surveys', *Implementation Science* 6, 15, http://www.implementationscience.com/content/6/1/15.

Parkin P. (2009) *Managing Change in Healthcare Using Action Research* (London, Sage).

Paton RA, McCalman J. (2008) *Change Management: A Guide to Effective Implementation*, 3rd edn (London, Sage).

Pearcey P, Draper P. (1996) 'Using the diffusion of innovation model to influence practice: A case study', *Journal of Advanced Nursing* 23, 4, 714–721.

Peng P, Stinson JN, Choiniere M, Dion D, Intrater H, LeFort S, Lynch M, Ong M, Rashiq S, Tkachuk G, Veillette Y. (2008) 'Role of health care professionals in multidisciplinary pain treatment facilities in Canada', *Pain Research and Management* 13, 6, 484–488.

Piderit SK. (2000) 'Rethinking resistance and recognizing ambivalence: A multidimensional view of attitudes toward an organizational change', *Academy of Management Review* 25, 4, 783–794.

Plastow NA. (2006) 'Implementing evidence based practice: A model for change', *International Journal of Therapy and Rehabilitation* 13, 10, 464–469.

Polkinghorne DE. (2005) 'Language and meaning: Data collection in qualitative research', *Journal of Counselling Psychology* 52, 2, 137–145.

Price B. (2008) 'Strategies to help nurses cope with change in the healthcare setting', *Nursing Standard* 22, 48, 50–56.

Price B. (2010) 'Disseminating best practice through publication in journals', *Nursing Standard* 24, 26, 35–41.

Prochaska JO, DiClemente CC. (1992) 'Stages of change in the modification of problem behaviours', *Progress in Behaviour Modification* 28, 183–218.

Pryjmachuk S. (1996) 'Pragmatism and change: Some implications for nurses, nurse managers and nursing', *Journal of Nursing Management* 4, 4, 201–205.

Qian Y, Daniels TD. (2008) 'A Communication model of employee cynicism toward organizational change', *Corporate Communications* 13, 3, 319–332.

Quattrone P, Hopper T. (2001) 'What does organizational change mean? Speculations on a taken for granted category', *Management Accounting Research* 12, 403–435.

Reed J, Turner J. (2005) 'Appreciating change in cancer services – An evaluation of service development strategies', *Journal of Health Organization and Management* 19, 2, 163–176.

Reid G, Kneafsey R, Long A, Hulme C, Wright H. (2007) 'Change and transformation: The impact of an action-research evaluation on the development of a new service', *Learning in Health and Social Care* 6, 2, 61–71.

Reid U, Weller B. (2010) *Nursing Human Resource Management Planning and Competencies* (Geneva, International Council of Nurses).

Reinhardt AC, Keller T. (2009) 'Implementing interdisciplinary practice change in an international health-care organization', *International Journal of Nursing Practice* 15, 4, 318–325.

Richens Y, Rycroft-Malone J, Morrell C. (2004) 'Getting guidelines into practice: A literature review', *Nursing Standard* 18, 50, 33–40.

Roberts P, Priest H. (2006) 'Reliability and validity in research' *Nursing Standard* 20, 44, 41–45.

Rogers EM. (1995) *Diffusion of Innovations*, 4th edn (New York, Free Press).

Ross F, O'Tuathail C, Stubberfield D. (2005) 'Towards multidisciplinary assessment of older people: Exploring the change process', *Journal of Clinical Nursing* 14, 4, 518–529.

Royal College of Nursing and Royal College of Physicians. (2006) *Acute and Multidisciplinary Working Policy Statement 16/2006* (London, RCN and RCP).

Russell CK, Gregory DM. (2003) 'Evaluation of qualitative research studies', *Evidence Based Nursing* 6, 2, 36–40.

Sackett DL, Rosenberg WMC, Gray JAM, Haynes RB, Richardson WS. (1996) 'Evidence based medicine: What it is and what it isn't', *British Medical Journal* 312, 7023, 71–72.

Sale JEM, Brazil K. (2004) 'A strategy to identify critical appraisal criteria for primary mixed-method studies', *Quality and Quantity* 38, 4, 351–365.

Saull-McCaig S, Pacheco R, Kozak P, Gauthier S, Hahn R. (2006) 'Implementing MOE/MAR: Balancing project management with change management', *Healthcare Quarterly* 10(Sp), 27–38.

Schifalacqua M, Costello C, Denman W. (2009) 'Roadmap for planned change. Part 1. Change leadership and project management', *Nurse Leader* 7, 2, 26–29, 52.

Schulenkorf N. (2010) 'The roles and responsibilities of a change agent in sport event development projects', *Sport Management Review* 13, 2, 118–128.

Scott T, Mannion R, Davies HTO, Marshall MN. (2003) 'Implementing culture change in health care: Theory and practice', *International Journal of Quality in Healthcare* 15, 2, 111–118.

Skinner D. (2004) 'Evaluation and change management: Rhetoric and reality', *Human Resources Management Journal* 14, 3, 5–19.

Soo S, Berta W, Baker GR. (2009) 'Role of champions in the implementation of patient safety practice change', *Healthcare Quarterly* 12(Sp), 123–128.

Stanleigh M. (2008) 'Effecting successful change management initiatives', *Industrial and Commercial Training* 40, 1, 34–37.

Stoller JK, Sasidhar M, Wheeler DM, Chatburn RL, Bivens RT, Priganc D, Orens DK. (2010) 'Team-building and change management in respiratory care: Description of a process and outcomes', *Respiratory Care* 55, 6, 741–748.

Tarling M, Crofts L. (2000) *The Essential Researcher's Handbook* (London, Balliere Tindall).

Tashakkori A, Creswell JW. (2007) 'The new era of mixed methods', *Journal of Mixed Methods Research* 1, 1, 3–7.

Tashakkori A, Teddlie C. (2003) *Handbook of Mixed Methods in Social and Behavioral Research* (Thousand Oaks CA, Sage Publications).

Thomas E. (2005) 'An introduction to medical statistics for health care professionals: Hypothesis tests and estimation', *Musculoskeletal Care* 3, 2, 102–108.

Tobin GA, Begley CM. (2004) 'Methodological rigour within a qualitative framework', *Journal of Advanced Nursing* 48, 4, 388–96.

van Bokhoven MA, Kok G, van der Weijden T. (2003) 'Designing a quality improvement intervention: A systematic approach', *Quality and Safety in Healthcare* 12, 3, 215–220.

van Meijel B, Gamel C, van Swieten-Duijfjes B, Grypdonck MHF. (2004) 'The development of evidence-based nursing interventions: Methodological considerations', *Journal of Advanced Nursing* 48, 1, 84–92.

Virani T, Lemieux-Charles L, Davis DA, Berta W. (2009) 'Sustaining change. Once evidence based practices are transferred: What then?', *Healthcare Quarterly* 12, 1, 89–96.

Wade DT. (2005) 'Ethics, audit and research: All shades of grey', *British Medical Journal* 330, 7489, 468–471.

Walsh K, Crisp J, Moss C. (2011) 'Psychodynamic perspectives on organizational change and their relevance to transformational practice development', *International Journal of Nursing Practice* 17, 205–212.

Weiner BJ, Amick H, Lee SY. (2008) 'Review: Conceptualization and measurement of organizational readiness for change: A review of the literature in health services research and other fields', *Medical Care Research and Review* 65, 4, 379–436.

Weiner BJ. (2009) 'A theory of organizational readiness for change', *Implementation Science* 4, 67, doi:10.1186/1748-5908-4-67.

Welch R, McCarville RE. (2003) 'Discovering conditions for staff acceptance of organizational change', *Journal of Park and Recreation Administration* 21, 2, 22–43.

Welford C. (2006) 'Change management and quality', *Nursing Management* 13, 5, 23–26.

Whiting LS. (2008) 'Semi-structured interviews: Guidance for novice researchers', *Nursing Standard* 22, 23, 35–40.

Wilson V, McCormack B. (2006) 'Critical realism as emancipatory action: The case for realistic evaluation in practice development', *Nursing Philosophy* 7, 1, 45–57.

Wilson V, Pirrie A. (2000) *Multidisciplinary Team Working: Beyond the Barriers? A Review of the Issues* (Glasgow, The Scottish Council for Research in Education, University of Glasgow).

Windish DM, Diener-West M. (2006) 'A clinician-educator's roadmap to choosing and interpreting statistical tests', *Journal of General Internal Medicine* 21, 6, 656–660.

Worden JW. (1991) *Grief Counselling and Grief Therapy* (New York, Springer).

World Health Organization. (2010) *Nursing Midwifery Services Strategic Direction 2010–15* (Geneva, WHO).

Wright S. (2010) 'Dealing with resistance', *Nursing Standard* 24, 23, 18–20.

Index